COLUMBUS AND THE NEW WORLD:
MEDICAL IMPLICATIONS

OceanSide Publications, Inc.

Providence, Rhode Island 1995

COLUMBUS AND THE NEW WORLD: MEDICAL IMPLICATIONS

Edited by:

GUY A. SETTIPANE, M.D.

Clinical Professor of Medicine, Brown University, Providence, R.I.

OceanSide Publications, Inc.

Providence, Rhode Island 1995

Contributors

Peter J. Bianchine, M.D.
Clinical Associate
Laboratory of Clinical Investigation
NIAID, National Institutes of Health
Bethesda, Maryland

Mark Blumenthal, B.A.
Executive Director
American Botanical Council
Austin, Texas

Sheldon G. Cohen, M.D.
National Institutes of Allergy
and Infectious Diseases
National Institutes of Health
Bethesda, Maryland

Manuel Luciano daSilva, M.D.
President, Bristol County
Medical Center
Bristol, Rhode Island

Jean-Claude Dillon
Institut National Agronomique
Chaire de Nutrition Humaine
Paris, France

Michael Fondu
Scientific Director
ILSI Europe
Brussels, Belgium

Clara Gorodezky, D. Sc., Ph.D.
Department of Immunogenetics
INDRE, SSA
Carpio, Mexico

Michael Grieco, M.D.
Professor of Clinical Medicine
Columbia University College of
Physicians and Surgeons
New York, New York

Marcos A. Ingelsias, M.B.A.
Mississauga, Ontario
Canada

Plutarco Naranjo, M.D.
Minister of Public Health
Ecuador

R. Allen Packer, D.V.M., Ph.D.
Microbiology, Immunology and
Preventive Medicine
College of Veterinary Medicine
Iowa State University
Ames, Iowa

Thomas A. Russo, M.D.
National Institute of Allergy and
Infectious Diseases
National Institutes of Health
Bethesda, Maryland

John E. Salvaggio, M.D.
Henderson Professor of Medicine and
Vice Chancellor
Tulane University Medical Center
New Orleans, Louisiana

Guy A. Settipane, M.D.
Clinical Professor of Medicine
Brown University
Providence, Rhode Island

OceanSide Publications, Inc.

Library of Congress Catalog Card Number 94-69156

Published by OceanSide Publications, Inc., 95 Pitman Street, Providence, Rhode Island 02906

Printed in the United States of America
ISBN 0-936587-07-5

DEDICATION

I dedicate this book to my parents and millions of other immigrants who followed Columbus's route from Europe to the New World. Their wilderness was a new culture, a new language, and severe working conditions. Their perseverance, hardship, and devotion to education imparted to their children liberty, creativity, and prosperity. They received and gave significant cultural contributions that helped to make America what it is today.

Guy A. Settipane, M.D.
Clinical Professor of Medicine
Brown University School of Medicine

Cover Photo: Columbus leaving Palos on his first voyage to the New World, 1492. Plate VIII from Theodor de Bry, *America,* Part IV, 1594. (Courtesy of the John Carter Brown Library at Brown University.)

COLUMBUS AND THE NEW WORLD: MEDICAL IMPLICATIONS

TABLE OF CONTENTS

Illustrations

FOREWORD

The practice of medicine and historical consciousness have a natural affinity. For it is impossible to be a physician and not have at least some awareness of predecessors and of a continuous Western medical tradition at least 2,500 years old. Any practicing doctor must see himself or herself as only one atom in this long record of human achievement, of human suffering, of folly and wisdom, all integral to the story of medicine.

Given this physician's inbred consciousness of the weight of the past, the appearance of this collection of essays should be no surprise. Precipitated by the observance of the quincentenary of Columbus's world-shattering voyage of 1492, the book looks at some of the biological and medical aspects of the "discovery," both scientific and social: disease, diet, the place of Jewish doctors in the new Iberian empires, Amerindian origins traced through blood and tissue types, the contribution of New World flora to the beneficial pharmacopia and to the dismaying list of known allergens.

What is distinctive about this collection is that it consists of articles written by doctors for doctors (and other interested parties). Most of the topics treated here have also been addressed at different times by professional historians, few of whom were medically trained; this is work, on the contrary, by physicians who have not been professionally trained as historians. The gain from such crossing of disciplines can be an expansion of horizons, the merging of scholarly literatures that had hitherto been quite separate.

Some of the issues treated in this volume remain basically unresolved and are still in need of as much learned opinion as can be mustered. Few subjects in the history of the Americas during the colonial period are as complicated and as difficult to reduce to any degree of certainty, for example, as that of the population count of Native Americans before Columbus's arrival and the effects of European diseases on that population. Eyewitness testimony is unreliable for various reasons. No witnesses were trained estimators of population size. Native American testimony was usually more impressionable than statistical. The pathogens raced ahead of Europeans, carried by Indians, so that when Europeans reached a particular Indian community, most of the damage was already done and the dead long buried. The very texts that serve as the only evidence we have, aside from archaeological interpretation, are often more flawed as sources than unsuspecting users might realize.

With regard to diseases, we have a driving desire to understand better what happened in that incredible and unprecedented historical moment when the "Oriental," (*i.e.,* the Amerindian), the European, and the African all came together for the first time. In the matter of new foods and drugs that resulted from the 1492 encounter, we are talking about massive contributions not only to the past five hundred years of human history but to the next five hundred as well. The anniversary of the European discovery of America is a good time to take stock of our dependence on nature's gifts, both those already realized and those yet to come—to come, that is, if we properly regard nature as a treasure and an expendable resource.

One can only wish in conclusion that this book will be a stimulus to active collaborations of physicians and historians in our common effort to tell and re-tell the story of early America.

Norman Fiering
Director and Librarian
John Carter Brown Library
Brown University

PREFACE I: 1450–1500 A.D.: THE WONDER YEARS

The 50 years from 1450 to 1500 A.D. represent the golden years of human civilization. These years were the last 50 years of the Middle Ages and the zenith of the Renaissance in Italy, with its nidus in Florence under the leadership of the Medici family. From Italy, the Renaissance movement spread throughout Europe, reaching its peak in the mid-seventeenth century.

Besides Columbus's remarkable discovery of the New World, many other great men and impressive accomplishments were present in this era. For example, in 1452 Leonardo da Vinci was born, and a year later Johann Gutenberg printed the 42-line Mazarin Bible. That same year the Turks captured Constantinople and killed Emperor Constanine XI, ending the Eastern Roman (Byzantine) Empire. The Turks' (Ottoman Empire) advance effectively cut off the Europeans', especially the Italians' (Venice, Genoa), trade routes to Asia. This blockade was a strong impetus for explorers to discover another route to Asia. The idea of discovering an alternate route was the main motivational factor for Columbus in discovering America. The Gutenberg press made written scientific information available more rapidly to scientists and explorers like Columbus (who owned several incunabula editions) so that they could continue their successful missions. This glorious period in 1452 also saw the completion of the Gates of Paradise doors at the Florence baptistry by Ghiberti. In 1456 precise drawings were made of Halley's comet, which appeared to present a portent of the golden period about to burst on civilization.

In 1461, Leonardo da Vinci became a pupil of Verrocchio. In 1469, King Ferdinand of Aragon married Queen Isabella of Castile, uniting Spain and laying the groundwork for a victorious war against the remaining Moors in Spain (Granada) and for subsequent support of Columbus's expedition to the New World. In 1473, the great astronomer Nicholas Copernicus, who gave the world the heliocentric theory of planets moving around the sun, was born. Columbus heavily relied on solar navigation, the North Star, and the compass in determining his position at sea. Scientists like Copernicus were important to him. Midway through this period (1475), the great Michelangelo Buonarotti and the English humanist and statesman, Thomas More were born.

In May of 1476, Columbus became a seaman on a convoy of five Genovese merchant ships owned by the Spinola and di Negro families heading for ports in the British Isles. In the Atlantic Ocean, Columbus's ship was attacked by French pirates and sunk.

In 1477, Columbus sailed to England as a merchantman on a Genovese ship leaving Portugal. While there, he supposedly visited Iceland on a British merchant ship. In 1478, Columbus married and lived in Madeira, an island 600 miles southwest of Lisbon. From there, he took trading voyages to the Azores and the Canary Islands, learning invaluable seamanship and wind conditions in those waters.

In 1482 and 1484, Columbus participated in voyages out of Lisbon to the Gold Coast of Africa, another valuable learning experience.

In 1483, Raffaelo Santi (Raphael), the famous Italian painter, and Martin Luther, the German Reformation leader, were born. One year later, Botticelli completed his famous painting, the Birth of Venus.

In 1485, King John II of Portugal turned down Columbus's request to sail west into the Atlantic Ocean to discover a new route to Asia. The Portuguese king was concentrating on financing expeditions along the coast of Africa.

In 1487, the Portuguese Bartolomeu Dias sailed around the southern extremity of Africa (Cape of Good Hope), coming close to finding an alternate route to Asia. This discovery, together with the excitement of further exploration of the sea, must have caused Columbus some anxiety that someone else would discover the secrets of the ocean and a route to Asia. It must have enhanced his determination to proceed vigorously with his own plans.

In 1487, Columbus's request for an expedition to explore the West Atlantic was turned down by King Ferdinand and Isabella of Spain. The monarchs were too busy fighting the Moors in Granada.

In 1488 King John II, after inviting Columbus to Portugal, again turned down his request for financing his expedition after much discussion with his advisors. In 1490 and 1491,

Columbus's request for expedition money was turned down by the Genovese government, King Henry VIII of England, and King Charles VIII of France.

In 1492, the Spanish conquered Granada, the last Islamic city on the Spanish peninsula, consolidating the monarchy of Ferdinand of Aragon and Isabella of Castile. This now allowed the monarchs to direct their attention to other matters.

One of these areas dealt with the idea of finding a new route to Asia by a young Genovese sailor with excellent persuasive powers, Christopher Columbus. After much debate, his plan of exploration was funded.

However, all the decisions of these reigning monarchs were not good. That same year, Jews were expelled from Spain, depriving Spain of many physicians, mapmakers, and other intelligentsia. The Jews were given 3 months to accept Christianity or leave the country. The Muslims were given a similar ultimatum. It is unknown how many used Galileo tactics of "sotto voce" acquiescence. That same year Martin Behaim of Germany constructed the first known world map in the form of a globe.

In 1493, Columbus returned to Spain and was outfitted with another expedition (17 ships, 1200 men, many plants, and livestock) and departed again for the New World.

In 1494, Charles VIII of France invaded Italy with a large army and succeeded in causing the first major outbreak of syphilis (imported from the New World) in Europe. That same year Nicolo Machiavelli began his bureaucratic career in the Florentine Chancellery, leading to the writing of his famous book, *The Prince.*

Also that year, a significant decision by Pope Alexander VI to divide the New World between Spain and Portugal by making the demarcation line in the ocean further west was signed in a treaty form.

In 1495, Leonardo da Vinci began the painting of the Last Supper; Michelangelo's Pieta was completed about 1498.

Columbus returned from his second voyage after 2 years, 8.5 months in 1496. He then departed on his third voyage to the New World in 1498.

In 1499, Amerigo Vespucci and Alonso de Ojeda left Spain and sailed to South America, making many discoveries. The New World was subsequently called America.

In 1500, Erasmus completed his famous book *Adagia,* a collection of proverbs.

That same year Columbus returned to Spain from his third voyage to the New World under arrest and imprisoned in irons. He was released, and his oratory skills enabled him to convince the Spanish crown once again to outfit him for his fourth and final voyage to the New World 2 years later.

The last 50 years before 1500 A.D. were truly magnificent years not only for the arts, science, religion, and politics but also for exploration. Portugal explored the coasts of Africa; Spain, Portugal, and Italy explored trade routes in the North Atlantic; and Spain authorized and financed Columbus to cross the Atlantic. The general spirit of the Renaissance, with its enthusiasm for exploring new forms of art and religion and an unquenchable thirst for navigation and scientific knowledge, must have inspired Columbus to daydream beyond the known boundaries and to pursue his dreams in a relentless manner. The constant wars, both large and small, waged by the European kingdoms must have had an inhibiting effect on the Renaissance, but all the kings and their armies were unable to stop the formation and activation of great ideas.

BIBLIOGRAPHY

Admiral of the Ocean Sea: A Life of Christopher Columbus. Morison SE. Boston: Little, Brown and Company, 1942.

Circa 1492 edited by Jay A Levenson, 1991, National Gallery of Art, Washington and Yale University Press, New Haven and London.

Columbus and the Age of Discovery, edited by Zvl Dor-Nev and William G. Scheller. 1991, WGBH Educational Foundation.

Encountering the New World, 1493–1500, Susan Danforth, 1991, The John Carter Brown Library, Providence, RI.

Europe 1492: Portrait of a Continent Five Hundred Years Ago, edited by Franco Cardini, 1989, Anaya Editoriale S.L.I., Milan.

National Geographic: Search for Columbus, Vol 181 (1): January, 1992.

The Columbian Exchange, Alfred W. Crosby, Jr. 1972, Greenwood Press Inc., Westport, CT.

The Literature of the Encounter: A Selection of Books from European Americana, Dennis Channing Laudis. 1991, John Carter Brown Library, Providence, RI.

The Timetables of History: A Horizontal Linkage of People and Events, edited by Bernard Gron, based upon Werner Stein's Kulturfahaplan. 1982, Simon and Schuster, Inc., NY.

The Log of Christopher Columbus translated by Robert H. Fuson, 1987, International Marine Publishing Company, Maine.

Guy A. Settipane, M.D.
Clinical Professor of Medicine
Brown University
School of Medicine

PREFACE II: COLUMBUS AND THE NEW WORLD: MEDICAL IMPLICATIONS

What we have attempted to accomplish in this book is to use modern medical knowledge to answer the many puzzling medical questions about diseases that devastated the Native American Indian (Amerindians). For example, why were the Amerindians so susceptible to European childhood diseases? Why were these diseases so severe as to cause millions of Amerindians to die? What were these diseases? How were these diseases brought over to the new world? How were they transmitted to the Native Indians? What diseases did the Indians give to the Europeans? What was the mechanism of disease transmission? What role did swine influenza play, especially since the Spaniards greatly depended on the swine for a source of fresh meat?

The new techniques of HLA tissue typing have enabled us to analyze present day Amerindians. Did the incorporation of new genetic material from the old world enable the Native Indians to fight infections better? What percentage of the present day Indian population have European, Oriental, and African HLA blood and tissue types?

In this book we have gathered some of the world's great medical specialists to help answer these questions. These specialists include health scientists from Mexico, France, Belgium, Canada, and the U.S.A. Three of the United States authors are from the National Institute of Health at Bethesda, Maryland. The opinions and conclusions from these experts are based on the best scientific knowledge available today.

Some topics have never been previously addressed. For example, Professor John Salvaggio's chapter on the exchange of allergens between the new and old world is very new. Dr. Gorodezky's chapter on genetic differences between Europeans and Native Americans using HLA tissue and blood types is in the very forefront of medical knowledge.

The controversy as to where syphilis originated is addressed by Dr. Greico and Dr. Naranjo. They hold opposite points of view. Early Spanish physicians and hospitals are thoroughly reviewed. These early beginnings make up some of the basic historical background of modern medicine in the Americas.

Some chapters were highly technical and were rewritten and simplified so non-medical readers can easily understand them. HLA tissue typing between Native Americans and Europeans was especially complicated and had to be modified into layman terms.

Hopefully, this book will serve as an important reference source for medical changes that occurred when Columbus crossed the sea to the New World.

Guy A. Settipane, M.D.

Acknowledgement: I wish to thank our publishing staff: Cynthia Burke, Candace E. Crowshaw, Michele A.L. Doherty, Carole Fico, Virginia Loiselle, and Joseph Settipane for their help in publishing this book.

Chapter 1

Introduction:
Columbus: Medical Implications

Guy A. Settipane, M.D.

The medical and biological effect of Columbus' discovery of the New World has been awesome. The new diseases that Columbus and those who followed brought to the New World caused the deaths of millions of Indians. Tribes that inhabited the Dominican Republic, which numbered about a quarter of a million, declined to about 14 thousand 20 years after Columbus's arrival, and in 1570 were further reduced to 125. Some estimates are that Old World diseases might have killed 95% of the native Indians. Santo Domingo had about one million Indians before Columbus arrived, but that number declined to 500 in 1548. Indians in Mexico City declined from 25 million to about one million (1605). In 1699, a German missionary was quoted as saying that "Indians die so easily that the bare look and smell of a Spaniard causes them to give up the ghost." Indeed, later settlers were amazed to see vast lands empty of Indians. Some Europeans were convinced that God had made room for people of the Old World. It is true that the Spaniards treated the Indians like slaves and put some to death to establish authority and discipline, but the number of these deaths, although not forgiven, were not great compared with the havoc brought by the European diseases.

The new imported diseases that caused so much death among the Indians were: smallpox, chicken pox, typhus, measles, diphtheria, whooping cough, influenza, malaria, yellow fever, and possibly typhoid fever (Table I). The Indians in turn sent to the Old World syphilis, the first of the Indians' revenge, and Chigger disease (Table II).

The accidentally imported European rat helped spread typhus and other diseases. Tuberculosis was endemic to the Indian population. Trichinosis was not described clearly by the Spaniards, but with the importation of European pigs, this disease probably also was brought to the New World. Malaria and yellow fever depended on the importation of specific mosquitos (intermediary hosts). When these mosquitos accidently were imported to the New World, the cycle was complete, and these diseases became rampant. The Europeans were carriers and the intermediary host, the mosquito, transmitted this disease from person to person. Typhus and malaria were not clearly mentioned in the old Spanish manuscripts, but healthy looking Europeans can serve as carriers. Quinine, a drug treatment for malaria, was an Indian medicine. It was originally used in a crude form from the bark of a cinchona tree that is found in the Peruvian Andes. Typhoid might have been responsible for the great killer epidemic among the Indians in 1545 to 1548. This epidemic was called "cololitli," and the cause was listed as unknown. Other epidemics were reported where the disease was unknown because of limited medical knowledge.

Most Indian mortality occurred during the first hundred years of contact with the Spaniards. Fourteen to seventeen epidemics were recorded between 1520 and 1600. The great killers were smallpox (1520 and 1521) (Fig. 1) and measles (1531 and 1532). However, some of the earlier reports might have lumped smallpox and chicken pox inasmuch as both have certain characteristics that may not be differentiated by lay people. For example, "pneumonia and pleurisy" were frequently reported to follow severe skin eruptions with fever. Chicken pox can cause chicken pox pneumonia producing severe cough, hemorrhage, and other lung complaints. The death rate was so great that one Spaniard wrote "they died in heaps, like bedbugs." The historian Alfred W. Crosby, Jr., states that smallpox devastated an Indian army that was about to annihilate Cortes and his soldiers. The leader of this Indian army (Cuitlahuac), nephew of Montezuma, died of smallpox

Clinical Professor of Medicine, Brown University, Providence, Rhode Island

TABLE I

Infectious Diseases from Old World to New World

Diseases	Remarks
Smallpox	These diseases killed about 90% of
Typhus	the Indians, who were extremely
Measles	susceptible. The deadliest dis-
Diphtheria	ease to the Indians was
Whooping cough	smallpox.
Chicken pox	
Influenza	
Typhoid	
Trichinosis	

along with a large portion of his army. If it were not for smallpox, Cortes and his conquistadors may have been annihilated but instead are given credit for a resounding victory.

The Spaniards were relatively immune to these Old World diseases because of hereditary reasons and previous exposure. Their weak European ancestors had died of these diseases centuries ago, and those who survived produced progeny that were relatively immune. In addition, they might have been exposed to their diseases in childhood when the disease is in its mild form. In Europe, only 3 to 10% of those who developed smallpox died, although a great majority of Indians who were so infected died. Other Old World diseases also took their toll on Indians. In 1585, Sir Francis Drake brought typhus from Cape Verde to the Caribbean Islands and Florida, causing a great epidemic that nearly exterminated the Indians. This epidemic had little or no effect on the Europeans. Except for whooping cough and diphtheria, most infectious diseases were not as visibly dramatic as the skin eruptions of smallpox, chicken pox and measles and were difficult to diagnose. It seems probable that some of these skin eruptive diseases might have been confused in the manuscripts written by the Spanish magistrates. Nevertheless, these relatively innocuous diseases for Europeans could kill persons with little or no natural immunity, such as the Indians.

It is now apparent that interbreeding among the Indians and the Spaniards saved the Indians from extinction. Of the Indians alive today, about 95% are Mestizos, a genetic mixture predominantly of Spanish and Indian. The early Spanish explorers such as warriors, bureaucrats, merchants, and clergy did not bring their women with them. As reported by Dr. Plutarco Naranjo, Minister of Public Health of Ecuador in a following article, it was the custom for Spanish men to choose the most beautiful Indian women to live with them. Once the women were pregnant, the Spaniard would simply select other women. From this miscegenation, many children were born. Statistically, a monogamous relationship between a young man and woman not practicing birth control would average about 12 children. We might guess that each Spaniard might have sired about 24 children. Appalled by the Span-

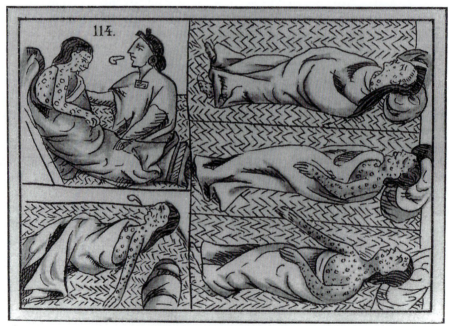

Figure 1. *Aztec smallpox victims in the sixteenth century. From Historia De la Cosas de Nueva Espana, Vol. 4 Book 12 circa 1565 (Courtesy Peabody Museum, Harvard University, Cambridge, Massachusetts).*

iard's promiscuity, the pious Queen Isabella in 1503 sanctioned this miscegenation by recommending and allowing Christians to marry Indian women. This official position of the Queen was ratified by Ferdinand V with the royal seal dated February 5, 1515. As the present day HLA and other tissue typing have revealed, it was the promiscuous Spaniards who appeared to save the Indians from extinction by sharing with them immunologically stronger genes.

It is not difficult to rationalize why the Indians envisioned the Spaniards as godlike figures to be obeyed, respected, and imitated. The Spanish soldiers wore armor, rode on great animals (horses), and carried weapons of great destruction: iron swords, muskets, and cannons. They were relatively immune to infections that killed hordes of Indians. They came from ships whose sails resembled the heavenly clouds. Indeed, Montezuma II fatally delayed to fight the army of Cortes because he believed Cortes to be the Aztec God Quetzalcoatl, who had returned to reclaim his kingdom. The Indians must have felt that any god whom the godlike Spaniards worshiped surely must be more powerful than their gods. Thus, it is easy to see why the Indians converted to Christianity in great numbers.

Syphilis was endemic among the Indians, and their natural immunity was considered very high, certainly much higher than was the Europeans'. The clinical symptoms were much attenuated in the Indians. The Europeans had never been exposed to syphilis. In fact, syphilis had not been described in any of the ancient writings dating back to the time of the Greeks, Romans, and Egyptian pharaohs. It never was described in the Bible. Unlike the Indians, the Europeans lacked natural immunity to this disease, and became very ill and died. Crosby states that physicians at that time agreed that it was a new disease among the Europeans (Table II).

Syphilis appeared in Spain in 1493, and it was thought to have been brought back by the crew of the Columbian expedition from Spain or by Indians Columbus brought with him. Ru Diaz de Isla, a Spanish physician, published a book in 1539 stating he had treated some of Columbus' men for syphilis. He called it "morbo serpentino," a sick snake, because he described the disease as hideous, dangerous, and terrible like a sick snake. He also stated that he had treated the commander of the Pinta, Alonso Pinzo, for syphilis. Reportedly, he was sick upon his arrival from the New World and died shortly thereafter. Dr. Ruy Diaz de Isla was a good physician because he noted that a high fever as that caused by malaria tends to ameliorate or arrest syphilis. In later years before the days of penicillin, this fever treatment was accepted by the medical profession, and it was shown to ameliorate syphilis. Also, Ferdinand, son of Columbus, wrote in the biography of his father that some of Columbus' crew had syphilis.

The term syphilis was first used in 1520 by Girolamo Fracastoro. The first large recorded epidemic of syphilis in Europe began in Italy. In 1494, Charles VIII of France invaded Italy with 50,000 soldiers of French, Italian, Swiss, German, and other nationalities. With the camp followers who accumulated as well as the rapes that occurred, a large portion of his army acquired syphilis. On return of his army to their respective countries, syphilis spread throughout Europe. It was then given the name the French disease because of King Charles's army, but the French called it the Italian disease named after the place where they contracted it. The Italians called it the Spanish disease because of where it originated, but it really was the Indian's disease or better still the Indian's revenge.

Some authorities believe that a mild form of European syphilis might have existed in the pre-Columbian days, but the mixing with the new Indian strain caused a virulent mutation of this disease. However, this appears to be unlikely. Europe was probably free of syphilis before Columbus returned.

The question arises as to why the Indians were relatively resistant to syphilis but extremely susceptible to the diseases listed in Table I. The answer lies in Darwin's theory of survival of the fittest. If Indian ancestors had encountered these European diseases, hundreds of thousands of years before Columbus arrived, then the susceptible Indians would have died at that time causing only those with greater immunity to survive and produce children. But this did not occur because the Indians remained isolated. In addition, the Indians contracted these Old World diseases essentially all at once (within one to two hundred years). If this process occurred naturally through thousands of years, one epidemic at a time, whole tribes would not have died essentially all at once, thereby risking complete annihilation of the Indian race.

TABLE II

Infectious Diseases from New World to Old World

Diseases	Remarks
Syphilis	Appeared in Spain shortly after Columbus returned to Europe (1493)
Chigger disease	Intensely itchy dermatitis caused by mite (chigger) larva
Others?*	

* Most new world diseases were not exported for various reasons: environmental factors, carriers, insect intermediary hosts, etc. were lacking.

That the native Indian genetic makeup is immunologically different from the European is manifested by studying blood and tissue types. Native Indians are almost entirely blood type O (95 to 100%). Europeans have blood type O 65 to 70% of the time. Seventy to 75% of Russians have blood type O, and 80 to 85% of Canadian Indians have blood type O. By the time the regions of the USA, Central and South America are reached, 95–100% of the Indians have blood type O. This may mean that the original tribe of immigrants that came through the Bering Strait seeded America with blood type O persons. A subsequent wave of immigration from Asia, thousands of years later began to dilute the blood type O Indians. This new wave of immigrants had reached the Southern Canadian border.

About 28,000 years ago, the Bering Strait, which is presently under 40 feet of water became dry as the sea water receded. The Ice Age had caused the water to be stored as glaciers at the North and South Pole allowing a transient strip of land to connect Asia to Alaska. For the first time ever, one or two tribes of Asians crossed over into the New World probably following herds of large game animals. Inasmuch as there were no humans in America, a rich source of foods existed because animals were not overhunted during this Ice Age as they had been in Asia. The new inhabitants thrived and multiplied. They slowly headed south seeding North, Central, and South America with blood type O persons causing the original Indians in America to have almost pure (95 to 100%) blood type O.

It is postulated that only a few Asian tribes made this trip through the land bridge of the Bering Strait. If there had been a mass migration, blood type B persons also would have crossed into America. About 15 to 20% of the Asian population contain blood type B persons, and some would have been included in the mass migration. This did not happen. American Indians are almost pure blood type O, providing evidence the migration was done in limited numbers. By chance alone, only one or two isolated tribes with blood type O crossed into America. The Bering Strait filled with water and the passage to the New World was closed about 10,000 years ago.

Several thousand years later when Europeans and Russians advanced to building sailing vessels, they reached the coastal areas of Alaska and Northeast Canada. The newcomers left genetic footprints among the Indians. Native blood was mixed with type B and A genes. Interior America as well as the non-Arctic regions remained almost exclusively blood type O. Nowhere in the world has such pure populations of blood type O people existed. Therefore, it is most probable that the seminal gene pool came from a small tribe of Asians.

The northeastern rim of Canada and all of Greenland have natives who have relatively more blood type A persons (25 to 30%) similar to the Norwegians (35 to 45%) and therefore may have been populated by the Norwegians. The northwestern rim of Alaska also has relatively higher blood type B natives (5 to 10%), similar to those people found in Eastern Russia (10 to 15%). This rim of increased blood type A and B persons probably occurred when fishermen crossed to America several thousand years after the original crossings. The blood type A and B genes have not been in America long enough to diffuse to the area presently known as Canada, USA, and Central and South America.

The practice of medicine in the New World was modeled after that existing in Spain during the period of Spanish colonization. An academic physician was required to have 4 years of study in a university leading to bachelor of art degree. The next 4 years were devoted to studies in medicine. The curriculum was lectures and commentaries based on ancient authorities as translated from Hippocrates, Galen, and Avicenna. To obtain a license to practice medicine, one had to continue the training for 3 more years (4 years for a surgeon) after receiving the doctorate degree. One then had to undergo examination by a strict bureaucratic government agency created in 1477 (called the Protomedicator), which examined physicians, surgeons, midwives, and apothecaries-spice merchants. Licenses were issued after passing the examination and payment of a fee.

This was a very rigid educational and training system for would-be physicians. Customary treatments were bloodletting, vomiting, purging, and sweating. Some of these treatments might have helped specific diseases such as bloodletting for congestive heart failure, vomiting for food poisoning, purging for constipation, and sweating (hyperthermia) for infectious diseases. However, if used indiscriminately, they would have nothing more than a placebo effect.

As bad as the practice of medicine was at that time, it suddenly became worse. In 1535, the Spanish crown issued instruction to require "limpeiza de sangre" (purity of blood) so that no one of Jewish or Moorish descent could officially practice medicine or enter universities. Because a great number of physicians in Spain were Jews or Moors, there was a tremendous shortage of physicians. The Protomedicator began licensing unqualified people as physicians to fill this void. Romance surgeons, those whose training was entirely by apprenticeship not by universities, began making a strong appearance in Spanish medicine. The strict control of the bureaucratic system of medicine began falling apart.

In 1545, there were only four licensed physicians in Mexico City. However, one of them was preparing to return to Spain because of overwork and poor health, and another was under investigation by the Spanish

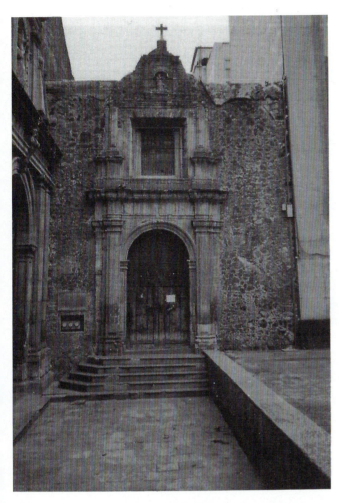

Figure 2. Hospital De La Purisima Concepcion and Jesus de Nazareno, First Hospital in America built in 1524. This is still and active hospital and has been operational for 468 years. (Photo courtesy of Clara Gorodezky, Ph.D.)

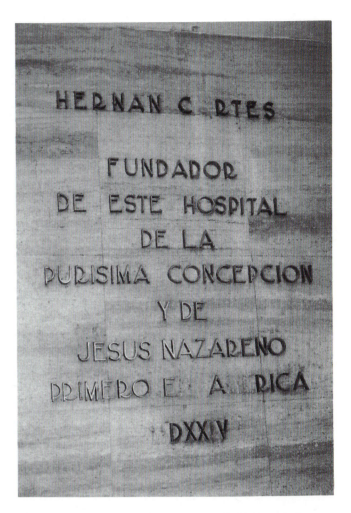

Figure 3. A plaque at the entrance of this hospital states "Hernan Cortes founder of this Hospital De La Purisima Concepcion and of Jesus de Nazareno, first one in America 1524." (Photo courtesy of Clara Gorodezky, Ph.D.)

Inquisition for use of sorcery (probably using Aztec herbs or other Indian methods). Of the two remaining physicians, one had a questionable diploma from a European medical school.

The University of Mexico was founded in 1551 and its medical school was established in 1578. The Spanish were health conscious and Queen Isabella of Castile decreed to the New World governors to "build hospitals where the poor can be housed and cured whether Christian or Indian." There were two types of hospitals in New Spain: a general hospital for all illness and specialty hospitals such as those for bone diseases and surgery.

Of all people, it was the Conquistador Hernando Cortes who founded the first hospital in New Spain in 1524 (Mexico City) called Hospital de la Purisima Concepcion and Jesus de Nazareno de Nuestra Senora (Figs. 2, 3, 4). This hospital was for the poor and sick, both Spaniards and Indians, but excluded patients with leprosy, syphilis, "madness," and "St. Anthony's fire." Cortes financed the hospital with his own personal funds, which must have been considerable after plundering the Aztec nation. By 1600, there were 12 hospitals in Mexico City, and by the early seventeenth century there were approximately 128 hospitals.

The Spaniards used the hospital to help convert the Indians to Christianity and for social education. This is similar to what the Spanish did to the captured Moors in Grenada. The hospitals were staffed by religious orders, such as the Franciscans and Augustinians. Many of the medical staff were immune to the infectious diseases because of past exposure. By today's standards, these hospitals were extremely ineffective in taking care of the sick. However, they did possess some effective drugs such as ipecac (induce vomiting), curare (causing muscle paralysis), cinchona (quinine), coca (cocaine), and cocoa (coca butter). In addition, coanenepilli roots had some antispasmodic effect. They also used avocado pits as an antidiarrhetic, extracts of agave leaves with honey as an expectorant, chili peppers and rhubarb as purgatives, hot chocolate as a laxative, and sarsaparilla

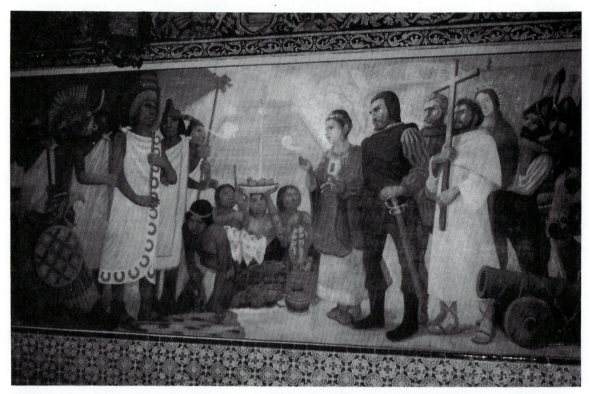

Figure 4. A mural in the first hospital of the New World with Montezuma (left) and Hernan Cortes with La Malinche (his Indian lover) standing in the area where this hospital was built (Photo courtesy of Clara Gorodezky, Ph.D.).

as a diaphoretic. In addition, they also used sapota fruits for asthma, cramps, and headaches. Most of these medications are at best only marginally efficacious.

There were some strong beneficial effects of these hospitals. They isolated the sick Indians with contagious diseases, they fed and gave them water (dehydration is a significant killer in febrile conditions), they provided them with clean sheets and offered sympathy. Some of the Indians were too sick to feed themselves and unable to obtain water if whole families or tribes became sick at one time. There was no one healthy enough to obtain food and water for the sick, and this contributed greatly to the death rate. These primitive hospitals did serve some of the basic needs of the sick.

Another important change that occurred in the New World's ecology was the importation of animals by Columbus including chickens, horses, donkeys, mules, cattle, sheep, goats, swine, and the great hitchhiker, the Old World rat (Table III). The European honey bee also was imported to America in those early years. In return, the New World exported to Europe the turkey, guinea pig, Muscovy duck, as well as the muskrat (for pelts) (Table IV).

Columbus made four trips to the New World. In his second trip in 1493, he arrived with 17 ships and 1200 men, a sharp contrast to his first voyage in 1492 when he arrived with 3 ships (Pinta, Nina, and the Santa Maria) and about 90 men. On his second trip (1493) he brought chickens, pigs, cattle, sheep, and goats. He also brought wheat, chickpeas, melons, onions, radishes, salad greens, grape vines, sugar cane, and fruit stones. "Kentucky's" blue grass was also imported to this country, and it proved to be very allergenic.

The history of the importation to American of pigs and horses is now legendary. The Spaniards were particularly fond of pigs. They seeded a male and female pig almost everywhere they landed. They knew that ships that crossed the ocean depleted their stores of meat. Crews from these ships then could harvest pigs on islands and mainland where they were left to forage and multiply. Indeed, the pigs proliferated. Crosby states that in 1542, Cabeza de Vaca in Rio de la Plata found a message from his predecessor that stated "In one of the islands of San Gabriel a sow and a boar have been left to breed. Do not kill them. If there should be many take those you need, but always leave some to breed, and also, on your way, leave a sow and a boar on the island of Matrin Garcia and on other islands whatever you think good so that they may breed." In 1539, DeSoto saw his 13 original pigs brought to Florida multiply to 700 in 3 years. An original two dozen pigs brought to Cuba multiplied to 30,000 in 16 years. There

TABLE III

Foods Imported from Old World to New World

Bananas
Barley
Cabbage
Chicken (Columbus)
Coffee
Cow (Columbus)
Dandelion
Goats (Columbus)
Grapevines (Columbus)
Lemons
Olives
Onions (Columbus)
Oranges (Columbus)
Peach (Columbus)
Pears (Columbus)
Pigs (Columbus)
Rice
Radishes
Sheep (Columbus)
Sugar cane
Turnip
Wheat

Note: Horses and large dogs also were brought to the new world by Columbus. Indians had a much smaller version of the pet dog.

TABLE IV

Foods Imported to Old World from New World

Avocado
Beans (Lima, navy, kidney)
Cacao (chocolate)
Cashew
Chili
Maize (corn)
Muscovy duck
Papaya
Peanuts
Pecan
Pineapple
Pumpkin
Squash
Sunflower
Sweet potato
Tomato
Turkey
Vanilla
White potato

TABLE V

Allergens from Old World to New World

Allergy	Source	Remarks
Stinging insect allergy	European honey bee	Affects about 1% of population, causes anaphylaxis
Feather allergy	European chickens	May cause asthma/allergic rhinitis
Egg allergy	Chicken vaccine, grown on egg broth	Hives/angioedema
Horse protein	Horses	Horse asthma and rhinitis
Milk allergy	Cows	Usually affects infants/children
Baker's asthma	Wheat flour	Occupational allergy
Grass pollen/ hay fever	Kentucky blue grass	Pollen allergy can cause hay fever and asthma

were pigs everywhere causing tremendous ecological damage to plants, snakes, lizards, and birds. The Spaniards had plenty of meat to eat with their living resupply depot, but they changed the ecological system of the New World forever.

From the Pleistocene Era, skeletal evidence of horses exists. However, there were no horses in the New World until the Spaniards arrived. Horses were left behind when the expeditions sailed back to Europe: others escaped. These horses found the New World grasses to their liking and multiplied rapidly. Indians captured and used these wild creatures to hunt and fight. They became mounted cavalry rather than foot soldiers.

Horses contributed to the demise of the buffalo because Indians riding horses were better equipped to hunt these animals, and the horses competed with buffalo in eating plants and grasses. Historians note that more species became extinct in the New World in the years after Columbus than occurred during the usual process of evolution over the last million years.

Animals brought from Europe also carried veterinarian diseases to the New World. These animal diseases are described by Dr. Parker in a later article.

The biological exchanges of plants from the New World to the Old World definitely favored the Old World. The New World received coffee, wheat, rice, barley, cabbage, turnip, sugar cane, lettuce, peaches, pears, lemons, oranges, and bananas as important foods

(Table III). In exchange, the Old World received the mighty corn and potato as well as tomato, pumpkin, squash, peanuts, pecans, and cashew as important food supplies (Table IV). The Irish, because of their accommodating soil, adopted the potato as a godsend and it also helped feed other European countries. The potato became so important that Marie Antoinette wore a potato flower as a corsage. It is presently estimated that now a third of plant food in the world are plants of American origin. The American plants took hold in European soil because they do not make great demands on the soil and do not compete with Old World crops.

This influx of American food into the Old World was a great factor in the population explosion that took place in Europe after the Columbus era. Despite the massive migration of people in later years from the Old to the New World (numbering in tens of millions), the population of Europe was not depleted but continued to increase. In other words, Europe gave up its surplus population, which was largely due to the increased food supply in Europe from imported American plants.

Special mention should be made about the tomato. It is a New World food brought to Europe. The Italians adopted it eagerly and blended it into their sauces. Today, it is impossible to think of Italian food without considering their red sauce. The tomato plant grew exceptionally well in Southern Italy, and this may be why the sauces in this region are primarily red; Italians in the Northern provinces have a cream sauce that reflects in part the old Roman cooking style.

Dr. Fondi and Dr. Dillon in a later article describe in detail the contributions of the New World food to the world supply.

ALLERGEN EXCHANGES BETWEEN OLD AND NEW WORLDS

The New World received several strong allergens from the Old World (Table V). One important source is the European honey bee whose sting can cause generalized hives/angioedema, bronchospasm, unconsciousness, and even death in about 1% of the general population. There had to be other native bees in North America, but the stronger European honey bee soon took over. The European bee was superior to native bees in collecting honey, but like other insects brought to America, it soon escaped its human caretakers and traveled about a hundred miles ahead of Spanish explorers. Reportedly, it was a warning to Indians, that the Europeans were coming.

Feather allergy is another source of a potent allergen accentuated by the European chicken. By the 1600s most chickens in America were European descendants. Feathers are used in down jackets, quilts, and pillows. Feathers were not entirely new to America. The American passenger pigeon, now extinct, reportedly migrated

TABLE VI

Allergens from New World to Old World

Allergy	Source	Remarks
Anaphylaxis	Brazilian Nut	Angioedema/hypo-
	Cashew	tension death
	Peanut	
	Pecan	
	Sunflower seeds	
Feathers	Turkey	Rhinitis/asthma
Others*		

* Tobacco is not an allergen but causes toxic reaction such as emphysema, chronic bronchitis, and lung cancer.

in packs of millions. Daylight turned to twilight as they flew overhead in great numbers for 3 or 4 hours at a time (Fig. 5). One might imagine the panic and allergy distress of the Indian or Caucasian who was allergic to feathers and suddenly found himself or herself under this great canopy of passenger pigeons. Many asthmatics and those with allergic rhinitis must have become symptomatic. These pigeons proved to be too docile and were killed by the millions when they alighted on bushes and low-lying trees to feed (Fig. 6). They soon became extinct because of the appetites of the Caucasians.

With the docile European chicken came the egg. Egg allergy is still troublesome in those persons who break out with hives/angioedema and other allergic symptoms after eating eggs. Another source of egg allergy is certain vaccines that are grown on an egg broth. Chicken and eggs as a food source and in vaccines are discussed in great detail by Dr. Sheldon G. Cohen from the National Institute of Health in other publications.

Horses and animals brought over on Columbus's second trip to America were the cause of horse asthma and rhinitis. Horse allergy is still present in certain sports enthusiasts, but it was a more common allergen in the days of horse-drawn carriages. Many old textbooks and research reports have documented horse asthma. Dr. John Salvaggio in an article that follows lists in great detail the allergens that resulted from the Columbus exchange.

The major allergens sent to Europe from America are peanuts, pecans, cashews, Brazilian nuts, and sunflower seeds (Table VI). All these foods are rich sources of protein and allergens. They cause severe allergies. Several anaphylactic deaths have been reported to peanuts and other nuts.

Although not a food but certainly chewable, tobacco (native to America) has caused a great deal of morbidity

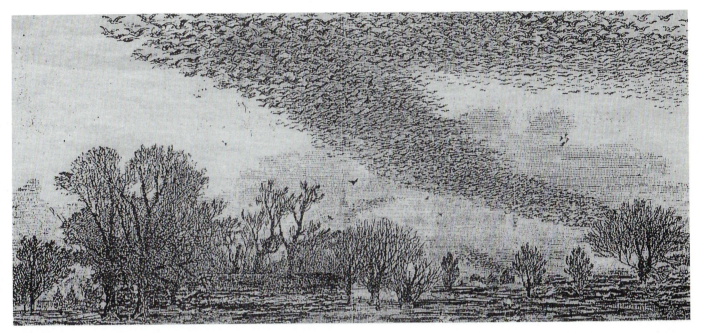

Figure 5. Migration canopy of passenger pigeons that reportedly was 200 miles long and thick enough to block the sun. They became extinct in 1907.

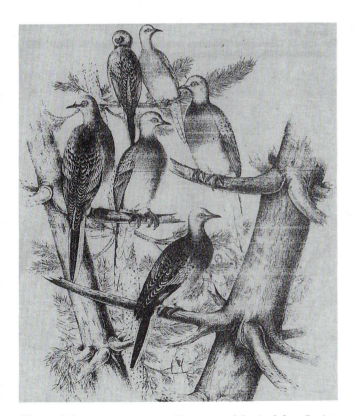

Figure 6. Passenger pigeons. (Courtesy of the Audubon Society of Rhode Island.)

and death among populations of the world. The devastating effect of long-time smoking habits have produced chronic bronchitis, emphysema, cardiovascular disease, and lung cancer. It has killed millions of people since 1492. If syphilis was the first revenge of the Indians then tobacco most certainly ranks as the second.

CONCLUSION

In summary, Columbus and early pioneers have changed the animal and plant life of America, Europe, and other parts of the world forever. It was the diseases that Europeans brought to America that killed millions of Indians. The major diseases were smallpox, measles, typhus, chicken pox, and influenza. In exchange, the Indians gave the Europeans syphilis and tobacco, both scourges of mankind. Genetically, the Indians were essentially a pure race of blood type O persons who crossed from Asia many thousands of years ago through a transient land bridge over the Bering Strait to America and who were extremely susceptible to European diseases. It is now apparent that interbreeding among the Indians and Spaniards saved the Indians from extinction. Modern-day tissue typing has shown that about 95% of the Indians alive today are Mestizos, a genetic mixture predominantly Spanish and Indian. It seems this interbreeding has conferred on the Indians immunity to help fight European infections.

Important animal and food imports to America were horses, cows, sheep, chicken, wheat, sugar cane, blue grass, and the European honey bees. Important exports to the Old World were corn, potato, nuts, turkey, tomato, cacao, and sunflowers. Many of these biological exchanges were significant allergens. Some authorities view Columbus's expedition as an ecological disaster. Others believe it was a great bonanza to Europeans because America's food plants (potato, corn, etc.) helped feed the great masses of starving populations in the world.

Early Spanish medicine was based on teaching of ancient authorities such as Hippocrates, Galen, and Avicenna. Rigid requirements and formal university training were set as standards. The expulsion of Jewish and Moorish physicians from Spain in 1535 created a marked shortage of physicians with only a few to spare for the New World. Nevertheless, the Spaniards built many hospitals in the New World beginning with the first one in 1524 in Mexico City. These hospitals were staffed by monks and priests. Although hospitals also were used to convert and control the Indians and adapt them to Spanish culture, they did provide food, water, isolation of the sick, and "clean sheets" for the sick. Efficacious drugs were limited, but physicians did possess ipecac (induce vomiting), curare (muscle paralysis), cinchona (quinine), coco (cocaine), and antispasmodics (roots). Other drugs were later developed from New World plants. In this compendium, an attempt is made to superimpose modern scientific knowledge with known historic facts about the Spaniards and Indians. In this manner, we are able to construct a reasonable understanding of what actually took place biologically and medically when the Old and New Worlds collided in 1492.

BIBLIOGRAPHY

Admiral of the Ocean Sea: a Life of Christopher Columbus. Morison SE. Boston: Little, Brown and Company, 1942.

Circa 1492 Levenson JA, ed. New Haven and London: National Gallery of Art, Washington and Yale University Press, 199.

Cohen SG. The chicken, in history and in the soup. Allergy Proc 12:47–56, 1991.

Cohen SG. Discovery and rediscovery. Allergy Proc 13:97–104, 1992.

Cohen SG. The chicken in history and in the soup II: Thank you Columbus. Allergy Proc 13:105–112, 1992.

Cohen SG, Mines SG. Variations in egg white and yoke components of virus and Reckettsial vaccine. J Allergy 29:479, 1958.

Cohen SG, Saavedra-Delgado AM. Through the centuries with food and drink, for better or worse V. Allergy Proc 11:89–96, 1990.

Cohen SG, Saavedra-Delgado AM. Through the centuries with food and drink, for better or worse VII. Allergy Proc 11:179–187, 1990.

Columbus and the Age of Discovery, edited by Zvi Dor-Nev and William G. Scheller. 1991, WGBH Educational Foundation.

Encountering the New World, 1493–1800, Susan Danforth, 1991, The John Carter Brown Library, Providence, RI.

Europe 1492: Portrait of a Continent Five Hundred Years Ago, edited by Franco Cardini. 1989, Anaya Editoriale S. L. I., Milan.

Medicine in the New World, edited by Ronald L. Numbers. 1987, The University of Tennessee Press, Knoxville, TN.

National Geographic: Search for Columbus. 181: 1992.

Plaques and People. William H. McNeill, 1976, Anchor Press/Doubleday, NY.

Seeds of Change, edited by Herman J. Viola and Carolyn Margolis. 1991, Smithsonian Institution Press, Washington and London.

The Columbian Exchange, Alfred W. Crosby, Jr. 1972, Greenwood Press Inc., Westport, CT.

The Literature of the Encounter: A Selection of Books from European Americana, Dennis Channing Laudis. 1991, John Carter Brown Library, Providence, RI.

The Log of Christopher Columbus translated by Robert H. Fuson. 1987, International Marine Publishing Company, ME. ☐

Chapter 2

The Role of Epidemic Infectious Diseases in the Discovery of America

Peter J. Bianchine, M.D., and Thomas A. Russo, M.D., C.M.

ABSTRACT

As the world prepares to celebrate the quincentennial events surrounding the discovery of the New World by Christopher Columbus in 1492, a particular interest regarding the influence of epidemic infectious diseases on the history of the conquest of America has emerged. Contrary to popular belief, it was not the European guns or fierce soldiers that conquered the native Americans, but instead it was the common childhood illnesses brought from the Old World by the European conquistadors. Diseases such as smallpox, measles, and typhus annihilated most of the American native populations. Devastating epidemics resulted throughout the New World. We will review the consequences of introducing new infectious agents into a nonimmune population, discuss the major pathogens that were imported from the Old World, and focus on how these diseases may have affected the aboriginal depopulation of the Americas.

As described in *The Ranks of Death: A Medical History of the Conquest of America*[1] by the late Colonel Percy M. Ashburn, a simplified overview of the European invasion of America is useful in tracking the effects of infectious diseases on the native populations. In brief, three major drives were taken by the explorers of that era into the Americas. The French invaded from the north and later down the St. Lawrence

From the Laboratory of Clinical Investigation. National Instituteof Allergy and Infectious Diseases. National Institutes of Health, Bethesda, Maryland

waterway over 1000 miles into the western plains. They proceeded south along the Mississippi to the Gulf and encircled the native Indian populations, effectively cutting them off from escape. The British formed a second drive that attacked along the Eastern coast at New England, extending from just south of the French settlements to Virginia along the southeastern seaboard. In combination with several small ventures from the Dutch and the Swedes, the British eventually invaded the entire eastern coast from Maine to Florida. The British tended to take up defensive positions, advancing in a slower contiguous fashion.

The Spaniards attacked from the south and formed the third major European drive into the Americas. Their preliminary ventures were under the direction of Christopher Columbus, or "Cristobal Colon,"[2] as he was known among the Spaniards. Spain controlled a vast empire in the fifteenth century, which encompassed areas extending from Holland, Austria, and Italy to the Americas. At the time the Spaniards were known to be formidable warriors and were universally feared throughout Europe. Their military strategy usually involved first establishing a preliminary base near the areas of interest that was later used for subsequent military expeditions. In the case of America, the island of Hispaniola, later renamed Santo Domingo, was established as such a base in 1492 and was used to consolidate military gains along the coast as well as plan deep forays to expand the Spanish Empire.

The most famous of the native populations in the Americas who opposed the Europeans were the Aztecs in central and northern Mexico; the Mayas in southern Mexico, Hondouras, and Guatemala; the Chibchas in Columbia; the Incas along the coastal slopes of Peru and Chile; and the Pueblos in southeastern America.[1]

In contrast with the French and the British. who concentrated their attacks on remote areas containing relatively primitive Indian cultures. the Spaniards aimed a massive military campaign at the heart of the Aztecs and the Incas. two of the most civilized and formidable Indian nations ever known. From 1492 to 1538 a series of Spanish expeditions moved west from Cuba to Florida and into the Mississippi valley. as well as south to Mexico. Panama. Columbia. and Peru. By 1580. these areas were permanently settled as part of the Spanish Empire. Of all the conquests of Spain. these campaigns were the most successful. By 1670. Spain signed a treaty with England establishing the boundaries of New Spain to include Panama to Venezuela. the West Indies to Charleston. SC. all areas west to New Mexico. and both the Atlantic and Pacific coasts. With the plundering of Central and South America by the Spaniards. the domination of the St. Lawrence and Mississippi valleys by the French. and the command of the east coast by the British. the European conquest of the Americas was virtually accomplished.

The geographical features of the territories taken by the Spaniards. the climate. and the density of the Indian populations all affected disease transmission. In contrast to the broad expanse of land in North America with diffusely scattered Indian tribes. Central America was a relatively narrow land mass. was easily accessible by both coasts. that allowed the Spaniards rapid access to virtually all areas by ship. Thus both geographic proximity and the high density of the Aztec and Incan populations permitted rapid and effective transmission of a variety of diseases (such as smallpox and measles) that are typically transmitted by direct person-to-person contact. The tropical climate of this region also supported the transmission of other infectious diseases such as malaria that required vectors (such as the Anopheles mosquito) not present in the more Northern climates.

Much of what is known today regarding the conquest of the Americas comes from the memoirs of two famous Spaniards. Bernal Diaz del Castillo and Bartolome de Las Casas. Diaz del Castillo was a retired and elderly soldier when he wrote *A True History of the Conquest of New Spain*[3] in 1576. Las Casas came to the new world as a layman in 1502. but he was so shocked by the oppression of the Indians that he entered the priesthood to fight for their fair treatment. He later wrote a five-volume collection called *Historia General de las Indias*.[4] now one of the few great sources of information from that era.

The obliteration of the native Indian peoples from the Americas was viewed in many ways by the Europeans of that time. The more religious groups from France and Spain deplored this action and grieved deeply for their loss: whereas. many of the British seemed to view the conquest of the Americas as a gift from God to His chosen people. Las Casas blamed the Spaniards for mistreating the Indians. for causing all their sufferings. and for their rapid disappearance. Antonio de Herrera. in his book *Historia general de los Castellanos en las Isla i Tierra Firme del Mar Oceano. etc.. en quatro decadas desde el ano de 1492 hasta el de 1531*.[5] tries to explain the rapid disappearance of the Indians in the region of Tabasco. Mexico:

> There used to be great numbers of Indians. but by reason of many diseases. and pestilences which they usually have in the province. they diminish greatly. because being sick with measles. smallpox. catarrhs. bloody flux. and great fevers. they bathe in the rivers without waiting for the diseases to subside. and so they die.[5]

A review of the post-Columbian medical history of the New World reveals that the first century after the arrival of Europeans and Africans was filled with multiple epidemics characterized by high mortality rates. The first documented epidemic began in 1519 and caused massive loss of life extending from New Spain (Mexico) to Central America and Peru.[6] From 1558 to 1560. smallpox arrived at Rio de la Plata in Central America. "killing thousands of Indians without touching a single Spaniard"[7] and later became one of the worst killers of that era. In Mexico. as many as 14 and in Peru as many as 17 epidemics were recorded between 1520 and 1600.[7] The horrific scenes were described by a German missionary in 1699 who said. "the Indians die so easily that the bare look and smell of a Spaniard causes them to give up the ghost."[8] Alfred Crosby. in his book *The Columbian Exchange*.[7] notes that the English were as efficient at disease transmission as the Spaniards and the Portuguese of that time:

> In 1585 Sir Francis Drake led a large expedition against Spain's overseas possessions. His men picked up some highly contagious fever—probably typhus—in the Cape Verde Islands and brought it along with them to the Caribbean and Florida. The malady spread to the Indians in the environs of St. Augustine. and "the wilde people ...died verie fast and said amongst themselves. it was the Inglisshe God that made them die so faste."[8]

From 1616 to 1619 the plague swept through coastal New England and "killed as many as nine of every ten it touched."[9] Clearly the most deadly of the early epidemics were those of the "eruptive fevers" such as smallpox. measles. or typhus. Because of lack of specific details regarding each disease of that era and the overlapping nature of the epidemics. the exact etiologic agent of any given epidemic is often misdiagnosed. In the chronicles of the sixteenth century. the Spanish word "viruelas" was often mistakenly translated as "smallpox" although it was intended to describe a general pustular skin rash. which may in fact have been chicken pox, measles, or typhus. Nonetheless, an overview of these specific diseases (see below) will outline the probable pathogenesis of these outbreaks.

VIRGIN-SOIL EPIDEMICS

The diseases brought from the Old World by the Europeans took a terrible toll on the aborigines of the New World. Local populations were so devastated by both infection and prostration that they could offer little resistance to their European conquerors. Several reports of incapacitating epidemics with many casualties greatly support the theory that these diseases decimated the aboriginal populations.[10] The majority of these diseases appeared to be unknown in the Pre-Columbian New World, including measles, malaria, smallpox, influenza, epidemic typhus, chicken pox, and diphtheria.[7-9] Epidemics that involve a geographically secluded population that has had no previous exposure to the pathogen in question are referred to as "virgin-soil" epidemics.[11,12] Such populations depend on effective neoantigen processing and immune surveillance to fight against novel pathogens, inasmuch as the nonspecific host defense mechanisms (e.g., complement mediated lysis or phagocytosis) are usually ineffective against virulent microorganisms. The concept that the native Indians were unusually "susceptible" to these pathogens was popularized after the time of the colonization of the New World. Recent studies analyzed the effects of both measles (rubeola) and a measles vaccine in a virgin-soil population of South American Indians, called the Yanomama.[13] These studies, which examined the tribe's first known contact with measles, indicated that the ability of the Yanomaman Indians to process rubeola viral antigens and form specific antibodies to these neoantigens was not significantly different from that of the oftenexposed Caucasian populations, nor was their mortality increased solely as a direct consequence of the disease. The presumed "constitutional" susceptibility to these pathogens may in fact reflect only excessive morbidity and mortality due to: (1) lack of nourishment during the illness, (2) lack of proper hydration during the illness, (3) ignorance of pulmonary toilet and excessive incidence of secondary bacterial pneumonia, (4) generalized terror and disorganization due to a lack of knowledge regarding the natural history of the illness involved, and (5) lack of available healthy persons to care for the ill because of almost simultaneous infection of large numbers of the population.

These observations have been made and recorded in several other virgin-soil epidemics.[14,15] In this study, given comparable care when ill and knowledge regarding the potential for surviving the illness, the death rates for virgin-soil Indian populations and repeatedly exposed Caucasian populations for measles were similar.[13]

These findings tend to dispute the theory that native Indians had a greater susceptibility to these illnesses than did Caucasians.

However, there is striking evidence that genetic factors can influence the mammalian resistance to a number of diseases,[16] including varicella,[17,18] malaria,[19,20] leprosy,[21,22] and typhus,[23] as well as influence immune responsiveness to streptococcal[24] or tetanus[25] antigens. Geneticists and molecular biologists thus continue to diligently search to identify human genetic polymorphisms responsible for specific disease susceptibilities. It is possible that specific genetic factors, in combination with these highly contagious infectious agents, were responsible for the demise of the aboriginal populations of the New World. The available evidence, however, suggests it is not necessary to invoke an increased host susceptibility to these pathogens as the major factor leading to these catastrophic epidemics.

THE INFECTIOUS DISEASES

The thesis that infectious diseases brought overseas by European conquistadors and explorers are in large part responsible for the aboriginal depopulation of the New World is supported in fact by many chronicles describing the ravages of epidemics that rapidly killed the native populations.[5,7,8] As previously mentioned, nonexistent or imprecise documentation makes it difficult to attribute specific pathogens to a given epidemic or to assess the contribution of the individual pathogenic agents in the overall demise of the native Americans. Nonetheless, we will describe the probable agents and speculate on their role in the conquest of the Americas.

Smallpox

The final battleground for variola (or the smallpox virus) occurred in Somalia in October 1977. Its eradication represents one of the greatest health care accomplishments of this century. Unfortunately for both the American aborigines of the early sixteenth century as well as for the seventeenth to nineteenth century Europeans, smallpox was one of their greatest scourges. Although smallpox was a new disease for the natives of the Americas, it had been present in Europe since at least the tenth century causing predominantly sporadic, nonlethal disease. Why this previously mild pathogen became one of the great killers in the Americas and later in Europe remains an intriguing mystery.

Smallpox is a relatively non-contagious disease with spread requiring intimate contact. There are no known animal reservoirs; therefore, infected humans are the sole source of infection. In the malignant form of the disease either myocarditis with resultant heart failure or extensive dermal involvement with severe sloughing and later complications are primarily responsible for the mortality rate of 15 to 45%.

The precise timing of the introduction of smallpox into the Americas is not known. An epidemic outbreak was described in Hispaniola at Santa Domingo, the original base of Columbus, in 1518.[4] This island was believed to be inhabited by approximately one million Indians, but by 1548 only 500 remained. Smallpox, either directly or indirectly, was no doubt responsible for many of those deaths. From there it spread to Cuba and other islands of the West Indies. Diaz del Castillo[3] reported the introduction of smallpox occurred into Mexico in May 1519. The Spaniard Narvaez sailed from Cuba where one of his black slaves acquired the disease.

He brought with him a Negro who was in the smallpox, an unfortunate importation for that country, for the disease spread with inconceivable rapidity, and the Indians died by thousands of it. ... Thus black was the arrival of Narvaez and blacker still the death of such multitudes of unfortunate souls, which were sent to the other world without having an opportunity of being admitted into the bosom of our holy church.[3]

After its arrival in Mexico smallpox spread quickly, in epidemic fashion, throughout the country with devastating results. Cuitlahua, the brother and successor of Montezuma, the Aztec emperor at the time of the arrival of the Spaniards, died from smallpox. The infection disrupted the organization and functioning of the Indian army defending Mexico at the time of the surrender of Mexico city in August of 1521:

The streets, the squares, the houses and the courts of Talteluco were covered with dead bodies: we could not step without treading on them, and the stench was intolerable. ... Accordingly, they were ordered to be removed to the neighboring towns, and for three days and three nights all the causeways were full, from one end to the other, of men, women and children so weak and sickly, squalid and dirty, and pestilential, that it was a misery to behold them.

By 1531 it was reported that the Mexican population decreased by a third;[26] smallpox undoubtedly was a major contributor to this decline. Pizarro's conquest of Peru began in 1532, but smallpox was probably first introduced from earlier costal explorations by the Spaniards or by contiguous spread from Mexico. The first epidemic probably occurred in 1519 to 1520, killing more than 200 thousand Peruvians, including Huayna Capac.[27] This was followed by a series of epidemics beginning in 1533, soon after the invasion. The Inca population in Peru was believed to exceed 10 million at its height. A census of 1548 to 1553 showed 8,285,000, and by 1791 only one million remained.[28] Smallpox was a major factor in their demise. Its spread was relentless with epidemics described in Brazil in 1563, into the next century in 1621 along the Amazon, in 1642 in Pernambuco, and in 1669 in Rio de Janeiro.[29]

Although death from smallpox was noted in the local Indian population soon after the French settlement of Canada in 1535, there were numerous epidemics from 1635 onward. The settlement of Plymouth, Massachusetts in 1621 might have been aided by an earlier epidemic in 1617 that was probably smallpox. The local population was devastated. Governor Bradford[30] wrote that the Indians were

not many, being dead and abundantly wasted in the late great mortality which fell in all these Parts about three years before the coming of the English; wherein thousands of them dyed.

Smallpox may have been introduced into the region overland from Canada, by English and French fishermen who had touched the coast during their expeditions, or by Captain Gosnold who landed on Martha's Vineyard in 1602. Governor Bradford[30] gives us a vivid description of the disease and its effect:

This spring also, those Indians that lived about their trading house there fell sick of ye small poxe, and died most miserably: for a sorer disease can not befall them: they feare it more than ye plague: for usually they that have this disease have them in abundance, and for wants of bedding and lining and other helps they fall into a lamentable condition as they lye on their hard matts: ye pox breaking the mattering; and running one into another, their skin cleaving (by reason thereof) to the matts they lye on; when they turn, a whole side will flea at once, (as it were) and they will be a gore blood, most fearful to behold; and they being very sore, what with could and other distempers, they dye like rotten sheep. The condition of this people was so lamentable and they fell downe so generally of this disease, as they were (in ye end) not able to help one another: no, not to make a fire, nor to fetch a little water to drinke, nor any to burie ye dead: but would strive as long as they could, and when they could procure no other means to make fire, they would burne ye wooden trayes and dishes they ate their meat in, and their very bowes and arrowes; and some would crawle out on all foure to get a little water, and some times dye by ye way, and not be able to get in againe.

During the 1630s smallpox raged up and down the St. Lawrence-Great Lakes region and killed more than half the Iroquois and Huron Indian federations.[31] By 1738, smallpox had killed as many as half the Cherokee nation and by 1760 more than half the Catawba tribes.[31,32] Smallpox ravaged most of the plains tribes shortly before the United States approved the Louisiana Purchase, killing more than two thirds of the Omahas and half the tribes between the Missouri River and New Mexico.[33] In the 1820s a "fever" now thought to be smallpox devastated the tribes along the Columbia River and progressed back over the plains in 1837 to kill half the Indian tribes located there.[34]

The precise reason why smallpox was so devasting to the aboriginal population of the Americas but barely affected the invading Spaniards, English, and French is and will probably remain unknown. We can speculate, however, on a number of possible explanations. Although the clinical manifestations of smallpox may be quite variable, it can be categorized into two forms that describe the severity of the disease (1) variola major and (2) variola minor. Variola major has a case fatality rate of 15 to 45%, whereas, variola minor less than 1%. This difference in pathogenicity is presumed to be secondary to a genotypic variation in the smallpox virus, but this has not been conclusively established. The clinical description and high mortality rates seen with smallpox when introduced into the Americas was unquestionably that of variola major. The problem with ascribing this as being the consequence of the introduction of the smallpox virus from Europe into the Americas is that variola major was essentially unknown in Europe at that time. It was not until the seventeenth century, about 100 years later, that the malignant form of the disease rampaged through Europe. A number of hypotheses can be forwarded, however, to explain this paradox.

The simplest explanation for the devastating effects caused by the smallpox virus in the Americas is that it was introduced into an immunologically naive population. This, of course, was true, but the problem with this rationale is that everyone who contracts smallpox is immunologically naive. Exposure to the various forms of the virus confers lifelong protection. Why then did contemporary Europeans contract the variola minor form of the disease and not variola major as seen with the aborigines of the Americas? Perhaps the answer lies in the timing of when infection occurred. In Europe smallpox was a disease of childhood. Adult infections were rare. Several infectious diseases have a asymptomatic or mild clinical course when contracted in childhood but are more severe when acquired at a latter age. Hepatitis A is generally asymptomatic or subclinical in the first decade of life and has an increasing propensity to cause clinical hepatitis with age. Epstein-Barr virus infection tends to cause the acute mononucleosis syndrome when the virus infects in adolescence or latter. Chicken pox is milder in childhood but can be severe and life-threatening when an unfortunate adult acquires it. It is possible that because the entire native adult population in the Americas was immunologically naive they suffered dire consequences from infection, whereas

Europeans were infected in childhood, a setting of perhaps milder disease. Problems with this hypothesis are: (1) Why did the malignant form of the disease devastate Europe about 100 years later? An interruption of the childhood infection cycle seems unlikely. (2) If infection was more severe in adulthood we might expect reports of epidemics from the Americas to mention a milder course in children. We have been unable to find such documentation.

An often-considered hypothesis for the devastating effects of smallpox and other infectious diseases on the native Indians is an increased genetic susceptibility to the effects of infection. This remains a possibility and may act in conjunction with other factors. However, there are a variety of other possible explanations for their demise from smallpox, and this possibility does not need to be implicated as the sole or likely mechanism. Remember, smallpox went on to ravage Europe 100 years after its introduction into the Americas, and it is unlikely that a gross alteration in the genetic makeup of Europeans occurred over that period.

When pathogens become more virulent one should consider the possibility of a genotypic alteration. With viruses, this most likely would occur through either point mutations or homologous recombination with a variant strain that has coinfected the same cell. It would seem quite coincidental for the European strain(s) of the smallpox virus, which at the time were causing variola minor, to mutate with their introduction into the Americas. A more appealing hypothesis is that the strain of smallpox that devastated the Americas came from Africa with the importation of slaves. We know little regarding the form of smallpox that was present in Africa at that time. Perhaps it was variola major. Somewhat against this theory is that the Spanish and Portuguese who had been contacting the African coast before the discovery of the Americas did not report contracting variola major. They may have been protected, however, by contracting variola minor in their childhood. We know the entire aboriginal population of the Americas was immunologically naive. Introduction of such a virulent strain would have predictably devastating results. A more outlandish speculation would be that the comingling of the European and African strains might have generated a "variola major" isolate that initially rampaged through the Americas and eventually made it back to Europe.

Measles

Rubeola (measles) is another of the acute, highly contagious eruptive febrile diseases that was brought with devastating results to the New World by the Europeans. Measles virus is transmitted by direct transfer of nasopharyngeal secretions or by airborne respiratory droplets to the mucous membranes or conjunctiva of susceptible persons. The illness is characterized by cough, coryza, fever, and a maculopapular rash. Recovery from infection is the rule, but respiratory or central nervous system complications may lead to death.

Many unexplained lethal epidemics of febrile eruptive skin diseases occurred in the early American settlements, and some of them were undoubtedly due to measles. Measles appeared to be less frightening to the Indians than the gruesome epidemics of smallpox, and measles came to be known as "la pequena lepra." Its appearance in the New World seems to be contemporary with or followed shortly after the introduction of smallpox. In 1530, Fray Toribio de Benavente Motolinia recorded measles as one of the "ten great afflictions of Mexico."[35] After the epidemic of "gran lepra" in 1519, a severe epidemic of measles extended from Mexico to Hondouras and Nicaragua, as described by both Herrera and Oveido in 1532. Oveido recounted that more than half of the population died of measles and other diseases that year.[35] Herrera also recorded a large epidemic of measles occurring in Peru simultaneously with a plague of locusts about 1540.[35] The Jesuit Père le Jeune described a series of dreadful epidemics of measles that occurred among the Canadian Indians in 1635.[35] Measles is often cited as one of the major killers of this era in the New World. Many of the fatal epidemics of eruptive fevers in early American history, however, are so poorly described that positive identification is impossible. Nonetheless, some of them must have been caused by measles. The extent of mortality directly attributable to measles is unclear. It received less attention than did smallpox in the literature of the time. It is unclear whether this is because of its being a less virulent pathogen and therefore less feared or because it was cosmetically less disfiguring. It is well documented that when measles is introduced into immunologically naive populations, it causes devastating results. This was seen in the Faroe Islands epidemic of 1846 where 6000 of the total population of 7782 were stricken, and more than 100 deaths were recorded. After measles was introduced to the Fiji Islands by H.M.S. Dido in 1875, the disease killed 40,000 of the 150,000 known inhabitants.[35] This variation in death rates is intriguing. The Faroe Island epidemic mortality rate was only 1.3% compared with the 27% rate in the Fijis; a difference comparable with that between variola major and minor. If both these rates are accurate, it suggests the effect of introducing measles into an immunologically naive population may be dependent on the characteristics of the given population and its societal makeup. If the higher mortality rate occurred in the Americas, measles would have been a killer of a magnitude similar to smallpox. Factors that may contribute to measles infection resulting in significant mortality are similar to those discussed above in virgin soil epidemics and smallpox. An adult susceptible population and perhaps genetic factors may play a role. In addition, disruption of societal structure resulting in inadequate supportive care can greatly exacerbate mortality from any infectious epidemic, especially if the population is recovering from or concomitantly affected by a smallpox epidemic. It is even possible to speculate that smallpox and measles infections occurred simultaneously or in close proximity in certain populations with a resultant synergistic increase in mortality. Between epidemics, measles almost certainly persisted causing endemic disease, as it does today. Although less dramatic, this mode of transmission will add a significant toll to society.

Epidemic (Louse-Borne) Typhus Fever

Classic epidemic typhus is a disease of humans caused by *Rickettsia prowazekii*, an intracellular gram-negative pathogen. Typhus is transferred from person to person by the bite of body lice. The lice acquire the organism in a blood meal and subsequently pass contaminated feces for 3 weeks until they die. When a human host scratches the site of a bite, he/she causes autoinoculation of feces into the epidermis. Times of war or natural disasters generate the conditions of overcrowding and lack of personal hygiene that foster the transmission of this agent. The Americas under seige was an ideal background for this infectious disease. Clinical manifestations include fever, chills, headache, and myalgias. A macular skin eruption occurs on approximately the fifth febrile day. Fever, vasculitis, prostration, and neurologic disturbances such as stupor, severe agitation, or even coma comprise the main features of the disease. Untreated, mortality is variable but can approach 40% under adverse conditions, with the elderly or debilitated most likely to succumb.

Typhus fever was known in the Old World as "jail fever," "ship fever," and "famine fever."[35] Typhus was introduced in New England and New France as "ship fever" and took hold throughout the New World, especially in Mexico and Peru where great epidemics occurred. A number of epidemics are recorded by both French and Spanish authors in which the natives suffered the passage of blood from the bowels and nosebleeds, consistent with typhus, typhoid, or dysentery. In 1637 there were reports of three priests, Chastellan, Dominique, and Jogues, who died of a "purple fever" suggestive of typhus. The esteemed Governor Bradford of the Salem Plantation also described many deaths due to an "infectious fever" in 1629 (which came from England with the ships passengers), again most likely due to typhus. By 1646, reports of an epidemic that killed more than half the Algonquin tribe owing to copious vomiting of blood were recorded.[35]

Again it is difficult to gauge the true effect this disease had on the New World. Its presence, however, is unquestionable. The setting was perfect for typhus to strike heavily. The natives were under seige from the Europeans and debilitated from a variety of infectious agents and poor nutrition. During World War I it was estimated that 30 million people were infected with typhus and three million died. It is easy to imagine that typhus was yet another infectious agent that caused significant mortality in the natives of the Americas.

Yellow Fever

Yellow fever is an acute infectious disease of short duration and variable severity caused by a flavivirus which was probably brought from Africa to the New World with the advent of the black slave trade. Human infection is caused by two distinct cycles of virus transmission, urban and sylvatic. Urban transmission cycles between humans and the *Aëdes aegypti* mosquito, whereas sylvatic transmission uses other mosquitoes (with lifelong infectious potential as a reservoir of the virus) that infect primates until another human victim is available. In mild forms, yellow fever occurs with the abrupt onset of fevers and headaches. More severe attacks progress to copious hemorrhages, anuric renal failure, jaundice, and delirium. The case-fatality rate is 20 to 50% when jaundice develops and about 5% overall.

An analysis of the introduction of African slaves to America is vital in understanding the introduction of yellow fever. Slavery was introduced into the West Indies around 1501. It has been speculated that along with the slaves in the slave ships came many diseases including malaria, yellow fever, and dengue fever. Like other diseases, yellow fever is an illness that depends on stagnant waters in which the vector mosquitoes breed. None of the investigations into the history of yellow fever ever conclusively proved the origin of this disease. However, several authors have weighed the evidence and concluded that yellow fever came to America from Africa on slave ships.[26] A French military surgeon named Audouard reported[28] in 1826 that the disease was selectively present and occurred with high frequency on slave ships from Africa but not on those ships used exclusively for carrying freight.

Oviedo[27] described the occurrence of yellow fever at Isabela, Santo Domingo, at the time of Columbus's second voyage:

And in the fort of Santo Thomas. . . . So they did not lack appetite to eat things very harmful to their health and fearful to see. From which and from the great humidity of the land many grave and incurable diseases followed in those who lived. And for this reason, those first Spaniards who came here, when they returned to Spain some of them who had come here seeking gold were of the same color as it; but not of the same lustre; for they became jaundiced and of the color of saffron and so sick that when or shortly after they were taken there, they died.

Oveido attributed the illness of Columbus's men to famine and spoiled food rather than to yellow fever. Medical accounts of these outbreaks were reported by Dr. Chanca, physician to Columbus's fleet on his second voyage, where he described that more than one third of the people had become sick. He believed the principle cause was the harsh passage across the sea and the differences in the land and failed to identify the cause as yellow fever.[29]

With respect to the conquest of America, yellow fever was not a major factor in the conquest itself, but it served as a by-product of the slave trade that caused severe human suffering and tragedy. The requirements for its spread, namely the flavivirus; the mosquito; the warm, moist climate; and the nonimmune persons were all present along the tropical coasts of America and the West Indies.

Malaria

Malaria is caused by the four species of *Plasmodium*: *P. falciparum*, *P. vivax*, *P. ovale*, and *P. malariae*. They are introduced by the bite of an infected female mosquito, usually of the *Anopheles* subfamily. Malarial parasites undergo a developmental period in female anopheline mosquitoes, which serve as the vector to infect humans. As the insect bites the human for a blood meal, it salivates and drools, allowing sporozoites passage into the body. Sporozoites then spread to human liver cells where they mature to merozoites or remain dormant as hypnozoites. Merozoites rupture from the liver cells to invade erythrocytes and to continue the cycle.

The characteristic malarial paroxysm consists of bed-shaking chills, fever, and drenching sweats. As the temperature rises, the patient feels headache, nausea, muscle aches, and often vomits. As the temperature falls, drenching sweats, rigors, and fatigue occur. Infection with *P. falciparum* can result in high parasitemia, and it is with this species that the majority of complications such as renal failure, pulmonary edema, or cerebral malaria occur.

There is no convincing evidence that malaria existed in any part of the Americas before the European conquest. Ponce de León, Pánfilo de Narváez, and Hernando de Soto were the early scouts who explored most of southeastern America and none of their recordings described great epidemics of malaria. None of the Huguenot or Spanish settlements in Florida or South Carolina mentioned any recurring febrile diseases of any kind. No clear indication of endemic malaria has been found until long after the introduction of African slaves. Once introduced, malaria spread slowly but surely. There are abundant references to malaria in the eighteenth century literature and personal letters of the period.

By the late 1700s to the early 1800s the entire Ohio and upper Mississippi valleys were infested with malaria. Many of the northern army posts such as Forts Brady, Mackinac, and Gratiot in Michigan, as well as others in Wisconsin, New York, and Ohio, reported large malarial epidemics.[35] Dr. S.P. Hildreth[36] recorded his personal views on these outbreaks and noted that malaria appeared only after the forests began to be cleared and the swamps were exposed to the sunlight. Therefore, the white settlers inadvertently created breeding grounds for the vector mosquitoes; a requisite for transmission of the disease.

The impact of malaria on the aborigines is unclear but at the least represents yet another infectious disease that contributed to their morbidity and mortality. The variety and continuing onslaught of new infectious agents undoubtedly contributed more significantly to the aborigines morbidity and mortality than did these agents individually.

REFERENCES

1. Ashburn PM. Chapter 2. In: Ashburn FD, ed. The Ranks of Death: A Medical History of the Conquest of America. New York: Coward-McCann, Inc., 1947.
2. Colon C. Memorial que para los Reyes Catolicos dio el Almirante Don Cristobal Colon, en la ciudad Isabela, a 30 de Enero de 1494. In: Navarette's Coleccion de Viages, 1494.
3. Diaz del Castillo B. Verdadera historia de los suceso de la Conquista de la Nueva Espana. In: Historiadores primitivos, Tomo II., by Vedia, 1576.
4. de Las Casas, B. Apologetica historia de las Indias. In: Historia de las Indias. Madrid: 1875–76, Vol 1–5.
5. de Herrera A. Historia general de los hechos de los Castellanos en las Isla Tierra Firme del Mar Oceano, etc., en quatro decadas desde el ano de 1492 hasta el de 1531. Madrid, 1720.
6. Dobyns HF. Andean Epidemic History. 1721, p. 514.
7. Crosby AW.: The Columbian Exchange: Biological and Cultural Consequences of 1492. Westport, Conn: 1972, pp. 31–63.
8. Stearn EW, Stearn AE. The Effect of Smallpox on the Destiny of the AmerIndian. Boston MA: 1945, p. 17.
9. Cook SF. The significance of disease in the extinction of the New England Indians. Hum Biol 45:485–508, 1973.
10. Jacobs WR. The tip of an iceburg: Pre-columbian Indian demography and some implications for revisionism. William and Mary Q. 31:123–132, 1974.
11. Dobyns HF. Estimating aboriginal American population: An appraisal of techniques with a new hemispheric estimate. Curr. Anthropology. 7:395–449, 1966.
12. Crosby AW. Notes and documents—Virgin soil epidemics as a factor in the aboriginal depopulation in America. William and Mary Q. 33:289–299, 1976.
13. Neel JV, Centerwall WR, Chagnon NA, Casey HL. Notes on the effect of measles and measles vaccine in a virgin-soil population of south american indians. American Journal of Epidemiol. 91:418–429, 1970.
14. Squire W. On measles in Fiji. Trans Epid Soc London (Sessions 1857–76 to 1880–81) 4:72–74, 1882.
15. Panum PL. Observations made during the epidemic of measles on the Faroe Islands in the year 1846. Biblio for Laeger, Copenhagen, 3R, 1:270–344, 1847. (English translation in Medical Classics: 3:803–886, 1939.)
16. Motulsky AG. Metabolic polymorphisms and the role of infectious diseases in human evolution. Hum Biol 32:28–76, 1960.
17. Lux SE, et al. Chronic Neutropenia and abnormal cellular immunity in Cartilage-hair hypoplasia. N Engl J Med. 282:231–236, 1970.
18. Harris RE, et al. Cartilage-hair hypoplasia, defective T-cell function and Diamond-Blackfan anemia in an Amish child. Am J Med Gen 8:291–297, 1981.
19. Allison AC. Protection afforded by sickle-cell trait against subtertian malarial infection. Br Med J 290: 1954.
20. Allison AC. The sickle and hemoglobin C-genes in some African populations. Ann Hum Genet 21:678, 1956.
21. DeVries RRP, et al. HLA-linked genetic control of host response to mycobacterium leprae. Lancet II:1328–1330, 1976.
22. Greiner J, et al. The HLA system and leprosy in Thailand. Hum Genet 42:201–213, 1978.
23. DeVries RRP, Van Rood JJ. Abstract tissue antigens. 10:212, 1977.
24. Greenberg LJ, et al. Association of HLA-5 and immune responsiveness in vitro to streptococcal antigens. J Exp Med 141:935–943, 1975.
25. Sasazuki T, et al. Association between an HLA haplotype and low responsiveness to tetanus toxoid in man. Nature 272:359–361, 1978.
26. Carter HR. Yellow Fever, An Epidemiological and Historical Study of Its Place of Origin. Carter LA, Frost WH, eds. Baltimore, MD: 1931, p.307.
27. Oveido GF. Historia general y natural de las Indias, Islas, y Tierra Firme del Mar Oceano, etc. 4 vols. Madrid: 1851.
28. Audouard M. Examen critique des opinions qui ont regné sur l'origine et les causes de la fièvre jaune. Paris: 1826.
29. Chanca Dr. Segundo viage de Cristobal Colon. In Navarette's Colleccion de viages, etc. Tomo I, 1494.
30. Bradford W. In: Davis WT, ed. History of Plymouth Plantation. New York:Scribner, 1908.
31. Duffy J. Smallpox and the Indians of the American Colonies. Bull Hist Med 25:328, 1951.
32. Washburn WE. The Indian in America. New York: 1975, p. 105.
33. Stearn EW, Stearn AE. The Effect of Smallpox on the Destiny of the AmerIndian. Boston: 1945, pp. 74–76.
34. Mooney J. The Aboriginal Population of America North of Mexico. Washington, DC: Smithsonian Miscellaneous Collections, 80, No.7, 1928.
35. Ashburn PM. In: Ashburn FD, ed. The Ranks of Death: A Medical History of the Conquest of America. New York: Coward-McCann, Inc., 1947.
36. Hildreth SP. Climate and early history of diseases in Ohio. J Proc. Med. Convention Ohio, at its Third Sess. Cleveland, Ohio: 1839.

Chapter 3

Epidemic Hecatomb in the New World

Plutarco Naranjo, M.D.

ABSTRACT

The American population developed, during thousands of years, free of epidemics that had been attacking Europe, Asia and Africa. The European and African migrations, after Columbus's first trip, produced an epidemic invasion of influenza, smallpox, measles, yellow fever, malaria, diphtheria, typhus, and other diseases that attacked the immunologically virgin populations and produced a very high mortality, with a diminution of the indigenous population of more than 90% in many places. According to historical evidence, the first epidemic was influenza, produced by suine strain of virus, immediately followed by smallpox. The Spaniards mated freely with the Indians producing a mixed race called the Mestizo, who were immunologically more capable of defending themselves against various viruses, bacteria, and parasites brought over from the Old World. Marriage between the races also was sanctioned by Queen Isabella (1503) and Fernando I (1515). With these new genetic immunologic defenses against infections, the Mestizo eventually made up the majority of the population of Indians in the New World.

For more than 30,000 years the American population from Alaska to Patagonia, had increased in number and remained isolated not only from Europe and Africa, but also from Asia, except, perhaps for some sporadic southern trans-Pacific contact. In this long period various epidemic diseases had sprung up in Asia, Europe, and Africa, caused not only by viruses, bacterias, and even parasites. Some of these are found documented in ancient Chinese medical textbooks as well

From the Academy of History and Academy of Medicine of Ecuador
Dr. Naranjo is Minister of Public Health, Ecuador

as in the Old and New Testament. Meanwhile, until before the arrival of the Spanish, Portugese, English, Dutch, French, Germans, etc., the American population had remained free from the attack of such epidemic diseases and, for that reason, they did not have the opportunity to develop any specific immunological defenses.

EPIDEMIOLOGICAL PROFILE OF SPAIN BEFORE THE COLUMBUS EXPEDITION

For several centuries before the American conquest, Spain had suffered consecutive epidemic waves of measles, smallpox, plague, and other contagious diseases. According to Guerra,[1] who had thoroughly studied this topic as well as had other authors,[2-4] the following chronology can be established (with reasonable accuracy) of first epidemics of diseases that resulted in havoc in the European population, especially in Spain. Smallpox appeared in Andalucia with the invasion of the Arabs from North Africa in 714. Leprosy appeared in Asturias in 923. Malaria, probably having come from Italy, appeared in Valencia in 1342. Plague appeared in the year 1348, spreading rapidly to various parts of the Iberian peninsula and causing many deaths. Of the flu or influenza, there are no documented reports as to how or where it originated.[5] However, it is known with certainty that there was a large epidemic in Florence (Italy), in 1357 which later extended throughout the Italian peninsula, registering a serious epidemic in Toscana in 1387. It is probable that from that time it propagated throughout the Mediterranean and reached Spain. Of course, in Spain this illness was very well known before 1492. Typhus appeared in 1489 among the soldiers who besieged Granada. Dysentery also appeared in 1489 among the soldiers that fought in Baza. Finally, diphtheria appeared in Granada, in 1530.[6]

EPIDEMIC INVASION OF AMERICA

Based on the clinical signs, particularly the cutaneous manifestations, there are documented reports concerning the first and following epidemics of smallpox. But the first viral outbreak, most likely, was not smallpox, but rather as Guerra maintains,[7] influenza, of the suine variety.

Bartolome de las Casa,[8] who left a detailed history of Columbus's trips mentions that, in the second trip, before starting the Atlantic voyage, in the island of La Gomera of the Canary Islands, the fleet obtained provisions not only of water, sponge cake, and other foods, as well as domestic animals: horses and mares, pigs, (the majority females), goats, chickens, etc., and plants and seeds, such as banana, sugar cane, and others. The pigs were transported in the bottom of one of the 17 ships that composed the fleet.

When the expedition arrived at the coast of the island, which in the first trip Columbus had named Española (Dominican Republic and Haiti), the admiral looked for several days for a suitable place to establish an urban settlement in the territory of the New World. Having chosen a place near a river, he ordered the unloading of 1200 men, together with the supplies and all the domestic animals that had been transported. He established the town of Isabela, in honor of the Queen of Spain.

According to Las Casas[8] and other historians,[9,10] who based their information on personal reports as well as on Columbus's own personal diary, a very few days after landing, there was a great epidemic outbreak that initially affected the Spaniards and later spread to thousands of inhabitants in the island. The disease was characterized by high fever, prostration that required bed rest, but with no cutaneous manifestations. Columbus himself got sick and was bed ridden for several days. This all happened in December 1493. The historians do not indicate the number of deaths, although they talk of a high mortality. It is known that in 1502 there were scarcely 200 survivors in addition to the few who returned to Spain in 14 ships from the second expedition after the unloading of the Spaniards.

Of the flu or influenza viruses that attack domestic animals such as horses and pigs, the most dangerous for humans are the ones that attack the pig or (suine variety), the same that in human beings has a high virulence of infection and produces a serious clinical picture. At times it has been called the flu or asiatic influenza, because it came from Asia, the place of origin of the pigs.

It is very probable, the first viral epidemic registered in the New World was influenza of the suine variety, which appeared as soon as the pigs were released from the bottom of the ship and made contact with the explorers. It could be assumed that although among the Spaniards (who were carriers of antibodies against the flu virus) there exists of a certain cross immunity between the various strains or varieties, there still was a high mortality. This was not the case with the indigenous population, who did not have any immune defense against the microorganism.

The appearance of black vomit or yellow fever was very rapid. It is possible that the disease could have been transported in Columbus's third trip, at which time the fleet stopped in Cabo Verde (Africa) in 1498 and after crossing the Atlantic, landed first on the island Trinidad and later on the island Española. But, as the presence of a vector is necessary, at least in this first phase, yellow fever did not spread as quickly as did the other diseases.

Probably one of the most significant demographic disasters of that era was due to smallpox. It is believed that smallpox came in a Portuguese ship that was transporting black slaves from Africa to the Caribbean; but it could have come from Spain as well, where the disease had existed for centuries. It is certain that in 1518 the first smallpox epidemic occurred among the Caribbean population. According to Alvarez-Amezquita,[11] a black man named Francisco de Eguin, arrived in Mexico in 1519, sick with smallpox, thereafter the disease spread throughout all the Aztec territory. By 1520 smallpox appeared in Chibcha region, which is the Colombian Caribbean coast, and began its invasion toward the south of the continent. In 1525 the disease had spread throughout the extensive territory of the Inca Empire. The emperor Huayna-Capac died after a few days of a feverish illness in the same manner as did more than 200,000 indians of his territories. Although Huayna-Capac had received a report of the presence of a white man in the coast of his empire, he did not get the chance to meet them, because the epidemic arrived before the Spaniard himself.

There are documented reports[11] of the first typhus epidemic in the Mexican territory in 1530, in which also occurred the flu epidemic of 1537.

The pigs transported by Columbus in his second trip to the Americas multiplied with surprising rapidity in the luxurient Caribbean islands, to the point that Las Casas,[8] mentions that the thousands of pigs that lived during his era, were descendents of the first group of animals. In the same fashion, the sugar cane and banana reproduced like weeds, for in the early part of the Spanish conquest, the Spaniards began to install sugar plantations for the production of compressed sugar, which sold at a very high price in Europe. But the cultivation and exploitation of sugar cane required manual labor. Labor they could obtain from the indigenous population was discounted because already 90% of the population had died, victims of the first epidemic. Thus it became necessary to import black slaves from

Africa, with whom also came diseases, such as malaria, that are characteristic of the tropical African zone.

THE DEMOGRAPHIC FALL

In the conquered territories the indigenous population entered a real state of slavery. The economic system, the labor system (in agriculture as well as in mining) and the alimentation system that the Spaniards imposed, with a limited diet and variety, meant premature death to the indigenous people and hence a demographic decrease. But more than these conditions and the physical abuse of which they were victims, that which violently decimated the American population was the successive epidemic invasions, which in a few years caused millions of deaths.

In the first years of the conquest, the first epidemics began in the Caribbean Islands where the ships made their first landing and later spread toward the coasts of South America and the Gulf of Mexico, where the population was annihilated by such diseases. There are appreciable differences of opinion among the historians about the size of the American population; there were those who considered it to be less than 20 million and to those, according to more recent studies, who estimate it to be 100 million. However, they are all in agreement that after Columbus's first trip the indigenous population was eliminated by 90%.

Table I summarizes the data of Cook and Borah[12] concerning the indigenous population in the island, Española, the same that 74 years after the first epidemic was practically extinguished and replaced by the black population from Africa.

The studies done concerning the demographic fall of Mexico, particularly those of Cook and Borah,[13] Table II, reveal that in the actual Mexican territory, in 1519 there most likely existed a population of approximately 25 million inhabitants, which had diminished to hardly a million in 1605, there remained just 40% of the population before the conquest.

Lipshutz,[14] using data from other authors was able to make an estimation of the South American Andean population. Table III, according to which, in 1532, the population was about 6 million inhabitants. But as Guerra[1] reminds us, the smallpox epidemic had extended throughout all the Inca territory in 1525, and as a result 7 years later, it would have cost the lives of hundreds of thousands or perhaps millions of inhabitants, not only in the Inca Empire but in general, in all the South American territory.

Although other studies exist concerning the rapid depopulation of America as a consequence of the epidemics, the previous examples cited are sufficient to appreciate the tremendous epidemiological impact the European conquest had on the American territories. The development of immunological defenses is a process that requires time and sacrifice of thousands and millions of people who succumb in the first infection.

TABLE II

Indian Population of Mexico after the Spanish Conquest*

Calendar Years	Years After	Total Population	%
1519	0	25,200,000	100.0
1532	13	16,800,000	67.0
1548	29	6,300,000	25.0
1568	49	2,650,000	10.5
1580	61	1,900,000	7.5
1595	76	1,375,000	5.5
1605	86	1,075,000	4.3

* *Borah and Cook and Lipschutz's calculation.*

TABLE I

Indian Population of "Española" Island (Dominican Republic and Haiti) after the Spanish Conquest*

Calendar Years	Years After	Total Population	%
1496	0	3,770,000	100.000
1508	12	92,000	2.450
1509	13	61,600	1.630
1510	14	65,800	1.750
1512	16	26,700	0.710
1514	18	27,800	0.730
1518	22	15,600	0.410
1540	44	250	0.007
1570	74	125	0.003

* *Cook and Borah's calculation.*

TABLE III

Indian Population of Andean Peru after the Spanish Conquest*

Calendar Years	Years After	Total Population	%
1532	0	6,000,000	100
1561	29	1,490,000	25
1571	39	1,470,000	25
1586	54	1,231,000	21
1591	59	1,300,000	22
1628	96	1,090,000	18

* *Lipschutz's calculation.*

THE EPIDEMIC INVASION OF ECUADOR

At the time of Spanish presence, the actual territory of the Republic of Ecuador, constituting a new part of the Inca Empire, was conquered less than a century before the arrival of the Spaniards to America.

The first epidemic of which there are reports[15-19] is of smallpox in 1525. Table IV shows the chronology of the principal smallpox epidemics, in the territory that was the Real Audiencia de Quito, actual Ecuadorian territory.

Because there are no clear reports concerning the first measles epidemic, which also appeared very early in the era of the conquest, it is questionable whether the death of the Inca emperor Huayna-Capac was really due to smallpox or measles. Nevertheless there are documented reports of measle epidemics since 1558.

Malaria probably appeared in the Ecuadorean coasts by the year 1600. According to the true historical information,[17] the treatment of the first paludal Spaniard with the dusts of cascarilla or quina bark was in the territory of Loja, southern Ecuador, in 1631.

Although typhus has been mentioned in earlier dates, there is documented information of its presence since 1611. The first cases of diphtheria were registered in 1612 with a high mortality. Yellow fever or black vomit appeared in the Ecuadorian coasts around the year 1700.

The mortality produced by the epidemics in the Ecuadorian territory was very similar to that which had occurred in other American territories. Costales,[20] found that the population in the island Puna, an important artesanal and commercial center and neighbor to the city of Guayaguil, had at the time of the conquest approximately 12,000 inhabitants. By 1690 it had been reduced to barely 12 families. Historian Juan de Velasco[15] mentions that the population of the area of Quito, with 80,000 inhabitants in 1589, after four epidemics was reduced to 50,000 and that there were some small villages that completely disappeared.

THE DEMOGRAPHIC RESURGENCE

Different from the puritan English, who came to America in 1620, for the purpose of creating a new country in which they and their entire family

---

TABLE IV

Chronology of Main Smallpox Epidemics in Ecuador*

```
1525+++
   1530            Sequence of epidemics
      1535         during the sixteenth century
         1558++
            1580
               1585
                  1587
                     1589++
                        1590
1611
   1612
      1645++           Sequence of epidemics
         1655          during the seventeenth century
            1657+
               1660
                  1669
                     1677
                        1692
1708
   1746               Sequence of epidemics
      1748            during the eighteenth century
         1759++
            1762
               1766
                  1783
                     1785++
                        1794
```

* The pluses mean more morbidity and mortality.

22

groups, bringing with them whatever possible material belongings, could freely profess and practice their religion, the Spaniards befriended the Western Indians in a plan of conquest; many with the sole dream of collecting gold and silver to return to Spain to enjoy this easily gained fortune. Thus, during the first years of the conquest, came young single men and married men, the majority arriving without their respective wives, a situation that encouraged immediate racial mixing. Some of them got married, but the majority took the most beautiful Indian women with whom to live. Not even the Catholic priests were exempt from this practice as relates Juan and Ulloa.[21] Even beyond that, Queen Isabella in 1503, sent instructions[22] recommending the support of the "Holy Mother Church that some Christians marry Indian women and some Christian women marry Indian men."

The official position of the Spanish crown was ratified by Fernando V with the royal seal dated the fifth of February 1515 and incorporated into the Compilation of the General Laws of the Indians of 1680.

With or without matrimony, the truth is that the Spaniards had no scruples against mixing with the Indians, giving birth to the Mestizo race that today populates Latin America. It is true, that although pure indigenous groups still exist, particularly in Ecuador, Peru and Bolivia, the majority relate to the Mestizo population. Within a few decades after the conquest, the Mestizo population of the New World became equal to the population of Spain. At the present time, only the population of Mexico is twice that of Spain.

What has been the immunogenetic influence in the demographic explosion? In what way did the genetic contribution of the Spaniards, carriers of immunological defenses against bacterias, viruses and various parasites, acquired over the centuries, contribute so that the American Mestizo population could develop their own biological defenses more easily and rapidly than the pure Indian? To what point did this genetic mixture affect the growth of the Mestizo population so that it soon surpassed in number the Indian population? Without a doubt the socioeconomic factor had a bearing, but is it possible to rule out the influence of the biological factors just mentioned in this accelerated population growth of the New World?

SUMMARY

The American population developed, during thousands of years, free of epidemics that had been attacking Europe, Asia and Africa. The European and African migrations, after Columbus's first trip, produced an epidemic invasion of influenza, smallpox, measles, yellow fever, malaria, diphtheria, typhus and others diseases that attacked the immunologically virgin populations and produced a very high mortality with a diminution of the indigenous population up to more than 90% in many places. According to historical evidences, the first epidemic was influenza, produced by suine strain of virus, immediately followed by smallpox.

The Spaniards mated freely with the Indians producing a mixed race called the Mestizo, who were immunologically more capable of defending themselves against various viruses, bacteria, and parasites brought over from the old World. Marriage between the races also was sanctioned by Queen Isabella (1503) and Fernando I (1515). With these new genetic immunologic defenses against infections, the Mestizo eventually made up the majority of the population of Indians in the new world.

REFERENCES

1. Guerra F. El intercamblo epidemiológico tras el descubrimiento de América. Manuscrito. Madrid, 1984.
2. Villalba J. Epidemiología Española. Madrid: Mateo Repullés, 1802.
3. Buoninsegni D. Historia Florentina. Firenze: Marescotti, 1580.
4. Astruc J. De morbis venereis Libri sex. Paris: Cavelier, 1736.
5. Saillant Ch. Tableau historique et raisonné des epidemies catharrales vulgairment dites la grippe; depuis 1510 jusques et y compris celle de 1.730. Paris: Didot Jeune, 1780.
6. López F. Breve reseña histórica de la difteria desde sus comienzos hasta el descubrimiento del suero diftérico. Madrid: Trabajos de la Cátedra de Historia critica de la Medicina, 1935.
7. Guerra F. La influenza, y no los españoles, acabó con los indios americanos. El Médico 159:47, 1985.
8. Casas B. de las. Historia de las Indias. Fondo de Cult Económ México, 1951.
9. Anglería PM. Fuentes históricas sobre Colón y América. Madrid: Impta S Fco de Sales, 1892.
10. Cieza de León P. La crónica del Perú. Madrid: Espasa-Calpe, 1945.
11. Alvarez-Amezquita J. Historia de la salubridad y de la asistencia en México. Secretaria Salub. y Asist., México, 1960.
12. Cook SF, Borah W. Essays in Population History. México and the Caribbean. Berkeley, CA: University of California Press, 1971.
13. Cook SF, Borah W. The Indian population of Central México 1531–1610. Berkeley, CA: University of California Press, 1960.
14. Lipschutz A. La despoblación de las Indias después de la conquista. América Indígena 26:229–247, 1966.
15. Velasco J. Historia del Reino de Quito. Quito: Casa de la Cultura Ecuatoriana, 1977–1979.
16. González Suárez F. Historia del Ecuador. Quito: Casa de la Cultura Ecuatoriana, 1969.
17. Arcos G. Evolución de la Medicina en el Ecuador. Anales de Univ Central del Ecuador, 306:967–1229, 1938.
18. Paredes Borja V. Historia de la Medicina en el Ecuador. Quito: Editorial de la Casa de la Cultura Ecuatoriana, 1963.
19. Naranjo P. El etnocidio epidémico en el Ecuador. Rev Ecuat Med 22:135, 1986.
20. Costales P. y A. Los aborígenes de la isla Puná. Quito: Supl Domin de El Comercio, 1984.
21. Juan J, Ulloa A. de. Noticias Secretas de América 2 vol. Madrid: Ediciones Turner, 1980.
22. Barceló de la Mora JL, Barceló Mezquita JL. Summ. Colombina. Diccionario Enciclopédico de Colón. Sevilla: Progensa, 1990. □

Chapter 4

Mechanism of Disease Transmission to Native Indians

Guy A. Settipane, M.D.,* and Thomas A. Russo, M.D.[†]

This chapter will discuss transmission mechanisms of contagious diseases to which native Indians were very susceptible, resulting in high death rates. The Spaniards were less severely affected by these diseases. This may have been due to Spanish immunity that was atavistic, in that great European plagues in the past killed many vulnerable individuals. Those who survived may have produced offspring who were genetically relatively immune. In addition, the early Spaniards were exposed to some of these viruses during childhood, a period of time when diseases such as chicken pox, measles, mumps, and others did not produce severe illness, but resulted in permanent immunity. Influenza virus was an exception. Why the aboriginal population of the Americas was so severely affected by a variety of infectious agents in contrast to the Europeans is discussed in greater detail in Chapter 11: "The Role of Epidemic Infectious Diseases in the Discovery of America."

SMALLPOX

Smallpox appeared in the new world near the end of 1518 or early 1519. According to Las Casas it began in Santo Domingo, killing most of the Indian population there. It then spread to Puerto Rico, where the Arawak Indians began dying in great numbers. Next it was seen in the Yucatan, where Bishop Diego de Landa recorded that "a *pestilence seized them (Indians) characterized by great pustules which rotted their body with a great stench...*"

Francisco de Aguilar, a former follower of Cortez who became a Dominican friar, stated, "When the Christians were exhausted from war (Cortez' battle with the Aztecs), God saw fit to send the Indians smallpox, and there was a great pestilence in the city." It lasted 60 days; and by that time, the city had been conquered by Cortes.

Crosby translated that "The street, squares, homes, and courts were filled with bodies so that it was almost impossible to pass." Reportedly with Cortez' army, there was a black slave who was suffering from smallpox, and this was the beginning of the great epidemic. Bernal Diaz del Castillo, an old Spanish soldier-historian, wrote that the negro represented "a very black curse (for Mexico), because. . . . the whole country was stricken with a great many deaths."

How could smallpox survive the long trip across the ocean without its being noted in the log? One possibility is that smallpox can be transmitted through clothes and other articles that were in direct contact with infected individuals. The black slave was probably given old clothes that had been stolen from individuals who died of smallpox. Some of the crusted material from smallpox sores

*Clinical Professor of Medicine, Brown University School of Medicine, Rhode Island Hospital, Providence, Rhode Island
[†]Head, Bacterial Pathogenesis Unit, Laboratory of Clinical Investigation, NIAID, NIH, Bethesda, Maryland

was probably still in the clothes. When the weather became cold on crossing the ocean from Africa to the New World, slaves were given old clothes to keep them warm. Unfortunately, some of these old clothes contained smallpox scabs. Therefore, this slave can not be blamed for beginning the greatest smallpox epidemic. It was the Spaniards who forced him to come to the New World, and it is possible that contaminated clothing given to him caused him to acquire smallpox. The invading Spaniards were less severely infected by smallpox at this time. The possible explanations for this vital biologic phenomenon are discussed in other chapters.

Presently smallpox has gone the way of the dinosaur; it became extinct because of smallpox vaccination sponsored by the World Health Organization. There have not been any outbreaks of smallpox since 1977. The only living smallpox viruses left are in laboratories, where they are safely stored awaiting future research that may be needed. For all practical purposes, the virus that killed millions of people since the beginning of time is extinct.

MEASLES AND CHICKEN POX

Measles and likely chicken pox are spread from droplets from nose, throat, and mouth of infected individuals in the pre- and early- erupting stages. These diseases are extremely contagious, with measles epidemics occurring in cycles of every 2 to 3 years.

White spots resembling tiny grains of white sand surrounded by a red areola area occurring opposite the first and second upper molars are called Koplik spots and are pathognomonic of measles. Besides the skin eruptions, these spots are associated with fever, coryza, hacking cough, and conjunctivitis. The incubation period is from 9–14 days. Measles was not a great killer of the Europeans, but it was reported as a great killer of Indians. It could have been transported across the ocean by two or three infected carriers in a sequential order.

The incubation period of chicken pox is longer than that of measles and is 14–21 days. Epidemic cycles occur every 3 to 4 years in the late winter and early spring months. Chicken pox is likely spread by infected droplets from the nose and throat. It is infective before and during the early stages of the skin eruption. Unlike smallpox, scabs are not infectious; therefore, it is not contagious through (third) non-infected persons or objects. The first skin lesions appear on the face and scalp and then spread downward, with the greatest concentration of lesions on the trunk. Laryngeal or tracheal vesicles may occur and cause dyspnea. Similar to measles, chicken pox virus may have survived the ocean voyage from Europe to the New World by two to three infected shipmates successively. In addition, shingles (herpes zoster), which represents an activation of the latent virus, can be infectious, causing chicken pox in nonimmune individuals. Although it rarely killed Europeans, chicken pox reportedly had a lethal effect on the Indians.

INFLUENZA

Influenza was thought to be another massive killer of Indians. The interesting fact about influenza is that some animal strains affect many animals (horses, pigs, birds, and humans). Animal reservoirs can significantly affect antigenic shift of the virus. The present-day example of this phenomenon is the swine flu that has been pandemic in modern times. Dr. Francisco Guerra, a member of the Department of History of Medicine, Universidad de Alcala de Herares in Madrid, suggests that the greatest mortality (of Indians) was caused by an epidemic of swine influenza. His theory is based on evidence from old Spanish chronicles such as Columbus and his physician Alvarez Chanda (the first medical graduate to practice medicine in America), Martyr Anglerius Fernandez de Oviedo, the well known Bishop Las Casas, Hernando (Columbus's son), and Herrera Tordesillas.

On his second voyage to the New World, Columbus landed on La Isabela, the first city of the New World, with 17 ships, 1500 men, and many domestic animals, including eight sows. A widespread epidemic began in December 9, 1493, the day after he landed. Reportedly, the men had no contact with the swine during the voyage and were exposed to them only upon landing in December 8, 1493. The short incubation period of this epidemic is consistent with influenza, which has an incubation period of 18–72 hours. Columbus and most of his men had immediate symptoms of high fever, chills, and prostration, symptoms also suggestive of influenza. There was a great mortality among the Indians who contracted this disease.

The Spanish were very fond of pork and placed breeding pairs of swine on various islands and the mainland. These pigs were allowed freedom to run wild and multiply. The Spanish intended that these wild pigs would provide fresh meat, a much needed commodity because their ships were on the high seas for several weeks and depleted their stores. Unfortunately, these transplanted swine may have been the source of an endemic reservoir of influenza viruses that caused periodic outbreaks among the non-immune Indians, thus causing a great mortality that was frequently associated with complications such as pneumonia.

TYPHUS

Epidemic (louse-borne) typhus fever was a killer of both Indians and Europeans. It is caused by *Rickettsia prowazekii*. Symptoms include a severe headache, fever of about 2 weeks duration, a macular rash, malaise, and vascular and neurologic symptoms. Typhus is transferred from person to person by the bite of body lice. Transmission is greatest in crowded unhygienic conditions such as in battle fields, armies, unclean ship conditions (*i.e.,* earlier times), and jail houses. In World War I, two to three million people died of typhus.

Typhus first appeared in Europe in 1490 when Spanish soldiers returned from fighting in Cyprus. In 1526 a

French army surrounding Naples had to withdraw in disarray because of a typhus outbreak.

Typhus was brought to the Indians by the early Spaniards. Transmission occurs when lice feed on individuals with either primary disease or the milder, recrudescent Brill-Zinsser Disease. This latter syndrome is characterized by an episode of typhus fever attributed to Rickettsial reactivation that can occur years after the initial episode. After body lice feed on an infected patient's blood, the Rickettsia infects the louse's alimentary tract. When the infected louse re-feeds, it defecates, contaminating the bite wound with infectious organisms. This disease can be quickly spread to an adjacent person by the louse vector, and it is facilitated by crowded conditions. Thus, the stage is set for an explosive killer epidemic.

YELLOW FEVER

Yellow fever may have been brought to the New World from Africa by the Spaniards. Conversely, it may have originated in South America. Nonetheless, the disease was first recognized in North America when the first epidemic of yellow fever occurred in the New World in 1648. This occurred in Yucatan and Havana. The mechanism of transmission of yellow fever is through a mosquito, *Aedes aegypti.* Once the mosquito became infected with this yellow fever virus (flavivirus), it becomes a carrier throughout its life span. Transovarian transmission of the virus occurred, resulting in progeny that are also infectious. Both mosquito and virus established themselves in the warm climates of the New World, as the mosquito was unable to propagate in temperatures below 72 degrees Fahrenheit. This mosquito breeds in small amounts of still water such as a water cask, cistern, and glass jars as found aboard ships. This means that infected *Aedes aegypti* could remain shipboard for weeks and months, causing a continuous string of deaths even in Northeastern ports such as Boston during the summer months. It earned the name "Yellow Jack" by English sailors since one of the main symptoms of this disease is jaundice. Other major symptoms are hemorrhages, (black vomit) and intense albuminuria. The usual incubation period is 3–6 days.

Upon recovery, patients were immune for life. This became the basis for yellow fever immunity before yellow fever immunization. Yellow fever caused many deaths among workers building the Panama Canal. Intensive mosquito-control measures were very helpful in controlling that Yellow Fever epidemic.

MALARIA

Most authorities agreed that malaria did not exist in the New World before the advent of the Europeans and the slaves.

Malaria is a protozoa infection characterized by recurrent fever and chills. Malaria parasites are found in the red blood cells and consist of four species: *Plasmodium* (P) *vivax, P. falciparum, P. malariae,* and *P. ovale.* They are transmitted from primate to primate, including humans, through the blood-sucking mosquito of the Anopheles family.

Africa is an endemic site for malaria. McNeil states that the malaria mosquito vector probably already existed in the New World. When infected Europeans and slaves from Africa arrived, the cycle became complete; and malaria, through Anopheles primate transmission, began a slow and progressive invasion of Indians and other primates (monkey, ape) throughout the New World. Malaria spread through South America and North America as far as Wisconsin, New York, and Ohio. McNeil states that in 1542, a Spanish expedition traveling down the Amazon did not lose any men from diseases associated with high fever, but they lost three men from Indian attacks and seven from starvation. Other early explorers of mosquito-infested tropics in the New World did not report diseases associated with high fever among the Spaniards.

One of the cardinal symptoms of malaria is recurrent high fever with "bed-breaking chills." The meticulous Spaniards who carefully chronicled these expeditions would have noted these intermittent high fevers and chills that are so suspicious of malaria. It is therefore likely that malaria was another disease brought to the New World by early settlers that added to the decimation and misery of the Indians. As a result, even in this day and age, no one dares to enter the forest of the Amazon without first taking antimalaria medications as a preventive measure.

SUMMARY

Smallpox, childhood diseases, influenza, typhus, yellow fever, and malaria are some of the major diseases brought to the New World by early explorers. Some of these diseases required the presence of an intermediate host such as body lice, mosquitos, and even swine. Other diseases were transmitted by soiled clothing. However, all of these diseases were endemic in the old world, and this meant that the early explorers had a relatively greater immunity to these diseases than the American Indians, who encountered them for the very first time. The effects were devastating.

BIBLIOGRAPHY

Plagues and People, William H McNeil, ed. Anchor Press/Doubleday, Garden City, New York, 1976.

The Earliest American Epidemic. The influenza of 1493, Francisco Guerra, Social Science History 12:3, 305, 1458.

Arrow of Disease Discovery, J Diamond, pp. 64–73, October, 1992.

The Columbian Exchange: Biological and Cultural Consequences of 1492, Alfred W Crosby, Jr., ed. Greenwood Press, Westport, CT.

The Role of Epidemic Infectious Diseases in the Discovery of America. Bianchine PJ, Russo TA, *Allergy Proceedings* 13:225–232, 1992.

Chapter 5

The Voyage of Columbus Led to the Spread of Syphilis to Europe

Michael H. Grieco, M.D., J.D.

ABSTRACT

The discovery of the New World by the Old World had a massive impact on subsequent events. It appears likely, but not certain, that the syphilitic epidemic in Europe may have been an imported affliction. It is impressive to appreciate how little was known in 1492 about infectious diseases and how much has been learned since the later decades of the nineteenth century. Syphilis represents the first major infectious disease for which discovery of etiology, development of a diagnostic test, and effective therapy were achieved, a major accomplishment of modern medicine.

It is difficult at the end of the twentieth century to appreciate the lack of understanding about disease pathogenesis present at the historic moment in 1492 which Christopher Columbus landed on an island in the New World. With regard to sepsis, three themes were prevalent and had emerged from Greco-Roman antiquity. One was that sepsis (putrefaction) and pepsis (fermentation) were two types of biologic breakdown, with and without a smell, that sepsis occurs in marshes, which produce fevers and other diseases and that sepsis produces animals by spontaneous generation.[1]

There was no real progress regarding sepsis during the Middle Ages and not until 1650 when Francesco Redi (1627–1697, an Italian physician and poet) decided to test whether sepsis really produced small creatures as Aristotle had said. Redi studied flies using his naked eye and won his battle against Aristotle. Soon thereafter the microscope was developed in 1675 by Leeuwenhoek, who managed to see some bacteria with his incredibly simple microscope. After that discovery bacteria were overshadowed by protozoa, which were easier to see and study. The scientific revolution in medicine had begun but well after Columbus had entered the New World.

Indians in the New World were characterized primarily by O blood type, suggesting limited heterogeneity of genetic constitution resulting from the limited migration across the Bering Strait during the Ice Age, occurring 15 to 25 thousand years before the birth of Christ. Infections prevalent among the Indians included tuberculosis, syphilis, parasitism, and dysentery. However, subsequent to Columbus they were exposed to devastating infections from the New World that led to reduction of the Indian populations from 50 to 90% in the Americas throughout the Western Hemisphere. Most Indians died from the white man's germs without ever seeing a white man. Epidemics of smallpox, chickenpox, measles, diphtheria, pertussis, and influenza proved to be devastating. Importation of pigs and mosquitos probably facilitated spread of trichinosis, malaria, and yellow fever.

A travel history constitutes an important aspect of inquiry when a specialist conducts an infectious disease consultation. We know too well the effect of travel on the spread of diseases such as influenza and HIV. So too did travel play a critical role in the spread of infectious diseases to the New World from the Old. However, one major disease pathogen apparently traveled from the New to the Old: syphilis. Thus the exporting of infection was not completely one sided. Syphilis showed up in Spain shortly after Columbus's men returned, and a lethal epidemic swept Europe within 5 years. A mild form of syphilis may have preexisted in the Old World but this is uncertain. When Charles VIII of France invaded Italy with 50,000 sol-

Director, R.A. Cooke Institute of Allergy and Chief, Division of Allergy, Clinical Immunology and Infectious Diseases, St. Luke's/Roosevelt Hospital Center, New York, New York Professor of Clinical Medicine, Columbia University College of Physicians and Surgeons, New York, New York

diers of French, Italian, Swiss, German, and other nationalities in 1494, syphilis spread among the troops and was disseminated throughout Europe after return of the troops to their individual homelands.

The population of Europe in 1492 was approximately 65 million, and 9 of 10 were peasants. Hardly 1 person in 20 could read, health was generally poor, famines often resulted from poor grain harvests, and rat-transmitted plagues were chronic. One in seven persons died of smallpox, and half of the newborns never reached the age of 15 years.

Medical therapy was essentially unchanged from the Roman period. Bloodletting was a common treatment. Food, housing, and possessions were very modest. Some peasants had a bench or a stool, but chairs remained rare. Martin Luther was 8 years old, Leonardo da Vinci 40, and Michelangelo a teenager. This was the world into which syphilis spread either because of European urbanization or, as seems more likely, because it was introduced from the New World.

SYPHILIS

Scientific Determination of Etiology, Diagnosis, and Treatment

It was not until the early decades of the twentieth century that three major discoveries thrust syphilis into the vanguard of medical science.[2] Metchnikoff successfully transferred the disease to chimpanzees in 1903. In May 1905 two German researchers, Fritz Schaudinn, a protozoologist, and Erich Hoffman, a syphilologist, found the spiral-shaped organisms in syphilitic chancres and other infected tissue. The organism was originally named *Spirochaeta pallida* and later renamed *Treponema pallidum*.

The discovery of the treponema was followed in 1906 by the development of a diagnostic test by August Wassermann and colleagues Neisser and Bruck who applied the complement-fixation reaction discovered by Bordet and Gengou to detect nonspecific nontreponemal reaginic antibody. He used fetal calf livers laden with *T pallidum* and subsequently extracts of uninfected beef livers and hearts. In 1909, nobel laureate Paul Ehrlich announced the discovery of salvarsan as a cure for syphilis. For the first time, a specific chemical compound had been demonstrated to kill a specific microorganism. Ehrlich called this 606th arsenical, which he had synthesized, a magic bullet. These developments in syphilis followed upon the germ theory of disease developed by Pasteur and Koch who identified organisms associated with other specific diseases such as tuberculosis, diphtheria, typhoid, and cholera.

From the sixteenth century well into the nineteenth, most physicians assumed that gonorrhea and syphilis were manifestation of the same disease. John Hunter's self-inoculation with urethral pus containing both *Neisseria gonorrhoeae* and *T pallidum* served to prolong this misconception. In 1837 Phillipe Record, a French venereologist established the specificity of the two infections through a series of experimental inoculations from syphilitic chancres. Dr. Record was also among the first physicians to differentiate primary, secondary, and late syphilis.[3] By the end of the nineteenth century the chronic manifestations of syphilitic disease was clarified. By 1876 cardiovascular syphilis had been clearly documented in the medical literature. By the early twentieth century, symptoms in one third of all patients in mental institutions were believed to have resulted from syphilis infection. The label "lues" comes from the Latin *lues venereum* meaning disease or sickness and was loosely applied to any venereal disease. It only become a synonym for syphilis at the turn of the twentieth century.

Before salvarsan (arsphenamine), syphilis had been treated with mercury, which was not curative. Induced fever therapy (malaria, heat box, hot baths) were apparently efficacious. Dr. Julius Wagner von Jauregg was awarded the Nobel Prize in 1927 for describing the use of malaria injections to treat neurosyphilis.

However, the treatments for syphilis had shortcomings. Arsphenamine was toxic, difficult to administer, and required an extensive regimen of treatment, sometimes for as long as 2 years. Only 25% of all treated patients apparently received the full complement of injections. The discovery of penicillin as effective therapy for syphilis in 1943 was the last milestone and established a regularly curative agent for this infectious disease.

Spirochetal Agents as Etiologic Agents[4]

The causal agent of syphilis is *T pallidum*, which belongs in the family Spirochaetaceae. Other mem-

---

TABLE I

Human Spirochetal Diseases and Their Etiologic Agents

Infecting Organism	Disease
Treponema	
T carateum	Pinta
T pallidum subspecies *pertenue*	Yaws
T pallidum subspecies *endemicum*	Syphilis, endemic (nonvenereal)
T pallidum subspecies *pallidum*	Syphilis, venereal
Leptospira interrogans	Leptospirosis
Borrelia	
Borrelia species	Relapsing fever
B burgdorferi	Lyme disease

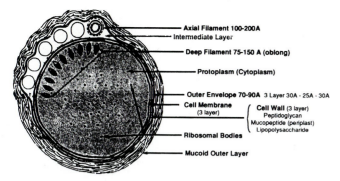

Figure 1. Cross section of a spirochete with six axial filaments.

bers of the genus *Treponema* that can infect humans are *T pertenue* (yaws) and *T carateum* (pinta). Other pathogenic organisms of the family Spirochaetaeceae belong to the genera *Borrelia* and *Leptospira* (Table I).

The organisms are slender, tightly coiled, unicellular, helical cells 5–15 μm (average, 10–13 μm) long and 0.09–0.18 μm (average, 0.1–0.15 μm) wide (Figure 1). The cytoplasm is surrounded by a trilaminar cytoplasmic membrane, a peptidoglycan layer, a delicate inner mucopeptide layer known as the periplast, an outer lipoprotein membrane containing lipopolysaccharide, and an amphorous outer layer. The end of the cells are tapered, and three fibrils are inserted into each end. It moves with a drifting rotary motion and usually has a characteristic undulating movement about the center of the organism.

The virulent treponemes, including *T pallidum*, cannot be cultivated *in vitro*. However, they have remained motile in highly enriched and specifically defined media up to 7 days at 35°C and up to 48 hours at 37°C. Rabbits are the laboratory animals most commonly used for maintaining virulent organisms.

Thus far no metabolic or structural immunologic or virulent marker differences between the pathogenic treponemes have been found, and the speciation rests primarily with the associated clinical illness.

Epidemiologically, spirochetal diseases follow one of two patterns. The treponemal diseases result from close skin-to-skin contact between humans, and there is no recognized animal reservoir of the treponemes that cause human disease. The remaining spirochetes (*Leptospira*, *Borrelia*) are zoonotic; that is, they have an animal reservoir in nature and infect humans via the direct or indirect contact of the latter with the animal reservoir.

CONCLUSION

The discovery of the New World by the Old World had a massive impact on subsequent events. It appears likely, but not certain, that the syphilitic epidemic in Europe may have been an imported affliction. It is impressive to appreciate how little was known in 1492 about infectious diseases and how much has been learned since the later decades of the nineteenth century. Syphilis represents the first major infectious disease for which discovery of etiology, development of a diagnostic test, and effective therapy were achieved, a major accomplishment of modern medicine.

REFERENCES

1. Majno G. The ancient riddle of sepsis. J Infect Dis 163:937–945, 1991.
2. Brandt AM. The syphilis epidemic and its relation to AIDS. Science 239:375–380, 1988.
3. Crissey JT, and Parish LC. The dermatology and syphilology of the nineteenth century. New York: Prager, 1981.
4. Tramont EC. *Treponema pallidum*. In: Mandell, Douglas, Bennett, eds. Principles and Practice of Infectious Diseases. New York: Churchill Livingston Inc., 1990, p1794–1808. □

Chapter 6

On the American Indian Origin of Syphilis: Fallacies and Errors

Plutarco Naranjo, M.D.

The first, and most severe, syphilis epidemic in history broke out in the Italian city of Naples between March and April of 1495. Most physicians of that period believed that this was a new disease. But those familiar with the history of medicine, including Leoniceno,[1] López de Villalobos,[2] and others, were convinced that though this particular outbreak was characterized by a spectacular and aggressive virulence previously unheard of, they were, in fact, dealing with a disease that had been around for a long time.

BACKGROUND

In the autumn of 1494, King Charles VIII of France decided to exercise his claim over the kingdom of Naples. To that end, he organized an army that included a large number of mercenaries from France, Germany, Flanders, Poland, England, Austria, Switzerland, and other nations. With a fighting force of 30,000 men, he set out from Lyon en route for Italy. The king's army crossed the Alps in October of that year and, soon after, reached the Duchy of Milan. For a variety of reasons, and as foreseen by Charles, the invading force encountered little or no resistance on its march, and entered Rome in triumph on December 31. The king organized a grand military parade through the city. In some neighborhoods of Rome the troops were even applauded. Pope Alexander VI (Rodrigo Borgia), fearing that he might be taken prisoner or fall prey to some other indignity at the hands of the invaders, took refuge in the castle of San Angel.

After negotiations with the pope, the unpopular Neapolitan king, Alfonso II, stepped down in favor of his young son who was unable to defend the city. Then, during the last days of January, 1495, the invading troops resumed their march to Naples. On February 22, Charles VIII led his men in triumph into that city. Subsequently, as was the custom among members of invading armies, they turned to pillage, theft, and rape.

THE BEGINNING OF THE EPIDEMIC

According to a number of famous Italian physicians of that period, especially Leoniceno[1] and Di Vigo,[3] a number of cases of venereal disease had been recorded both in Naples and in Rome prior to the arrival of the invading force.

In March and April of 1495, Charles VIII's men became seriously ill with a contagious disease characterized by fever, hard ulcerations on the penis, buboes in the groin area, and varied and fetid skin ulcerations on other parts of the body, especially the face. The soldiers of the French army called the disease *morbus napolitanus* (the Naples, or Neapolitan, disease), whereas the Neapolitans, who believed that the illness had been brought by the French, called it the *morbus gallicus* (the French disease).

We know, from historical documents, that central Italy, and, especially, Naples and the surrounding areas, had long been infamous for the corruption and licentiousness of its inhabitants. This was especially true during the time of the emperors. In one of his works, Marcus Tullius Cicero[4] described the profligate customs of residents of the province of Campania and, above all, of the city of Capua, near Naples, calling the site a *domicilium impudicitiae*, that is, the home of shamelessness.

Member of the Academies of Medicine and History of Ecuador, Quito, Ecuador, and Minister of Public Health, Ecuador.

The poet Horace,[5] celebrating the triumph of Augustus in one of his odes, invites his listeners to raise a cup of wine in honor of the emperor who "has saved Rome, whereas that queen (Cleopatra) was intent upon the ruin of the capital and the death of the empire by means of the spread of a fetid disease by members of a vile and shameful army." The same poet, in a reference to the face of Mesio, disfigured by scars, called the sickness the disease of Campania.

Another famous poet, Ovid,[8] speaks, in one of his verses, about the licentiousness of Rome in these words: "a mortal lues has contaminated the air of Lacio."

In Italy and especially Naples, prostitution was not only tolerated but even, in some ways, encouraged; thus, in cities like Naples, Rome, and Venice, the number of prostitutes was on the rise.[7]

Charles VIII's army was accompanied by servants as well as hundreds of prostitutes, as many as 500, according to some authors.[8]

A mercenary army has little in common with modern, well-disciplined troops trained in the arts of war. One can imagine the havoc wreaked by more than 30,000 men who have taken over a city where licentious acts and sex-for-sale are thought to be acceptable. During this period in Naples, the conditions were ideal for a venereal outbreak of epidemic proportions: overcrowding, promiscuity, prostitution. Even if, under such conditions, only a handful of soldiers carried the disease at the beginning, these would have passed it to the prostitutes who, in turn, would have spread the disease to a host of others since, no matter how many women were available, they were servicing an army of 30,000 and, thus, each most certainly had multiple contacts.

Because the disease was so virulent, it was fatal for some soldiers—exact figures are not available—and even more returned home carrying the disease with them.

THE SPREAD OF THE EPIDEMIC

As a result of the large number of soldiers affected, as well as for tactical reasons, Charles VIII decided to return to France immediately. The retreat began on May 22. On reaching Lyon, the troops were demobilized and the mercenaries returned to their countries of origin.

The return march of the invading army left a trail of syphilis from Naples to the north of Italy. On July 6, Italian troops offered their first show of resistance, which led to the only battle of the campaign; the Italians were easily defeated. Physician Marcellus Cumanus[9] wrote that, among the defeated troops in Fornobo, he treated patients affected by *morbus napolitanus*; this indicates that the Italian population, both military and civil, was infected and involved in the spread of the contagious disease.

From the end of 1495 to the beginning of 1496, a venereal disease called *morbus gallicus* spread to Germany, Holland, England, Austria, Switzerland, Spain, and, later, to Hungary, the Scandinavian countries, Russia, and finally, to Asia, including India, China, and Japan. Much has been written about the spread of syphilis throughout the world[10, 11] and thus this information need not be repeated in detail here.

It is worth noting that the spread of the disease was so rapid and alarming that authorities in a number of cities were obliged to take preventive measures and, in some cases, impose drastic sanctions. For example, the Parliament of Paris ordered all those who suffered from a venereal disease to abandon the city immediately or be thrown into the river. Holcomb[10] mentions this edict and states that it was issued in March, 1493, whereas Allen-Pusey and others state that it was issued in 1496; the latter date is most certainly the correct one. In 1496, the authorities of the French city of Aix dictated ordinances that included preventive measures. These forbade barbers from shaving the sick in order to prevent the spread of the disease. In that same year, on August 7, the Diet of Worms promulgated the *edictus in blasfemus*, and Emperor Maximilian ordered that preventive measures be taken against what he called "demoniacal pustules." Between 1496 and 1497, the cities of Nuremberg and Aberdeen (Scotland) also approved dispositions similar to the ones already mentioned.

THE FIRST PUBLISHED WORK DESCRIBING SYPHILIS

It appears that the first treatise dealing with this "new" disease is a work by Joseph Grünpeck,[12] published during the final months of 1496. The work, published in Ausburg in two editions, was entitled *Ein hubscher Tractat von dem ursprung des Bosen Franzos*, in German and, *Tractatus de Origene pestilentiali Scorra sive Mala de Franzos* (*Treatise on the Origins of a Plague Known as the French Disease*), in Latin.

Two brief works that appeared in the same year merit mention. In his work, Theodorico Ulsenio, a physician from Nuremberg, claimed that the disease had been caused by the conjunction of Jupiter, Saturn, and Mars (Fig. 1). His pamphlet included an excellent drawing by the famous artist Albrecht Durer, of a patient with skin lesions. Konrad Schelling (see Holcomb[10]) published a short study in which he referred to this new disease as "pustules" (*In pustulis malas morbum quem malun de Francia vulgatus appellat, quae sunt de genere formicarum*, 1496). The following year, Hans Widemann wrote *De pustulis et morbo qui vulgo mal de franzos appellatur*.

Among the many names invested to identify the disease, syphilis was the one that finally prevailed. Though the term was coined by Fracastoro in 1530, it

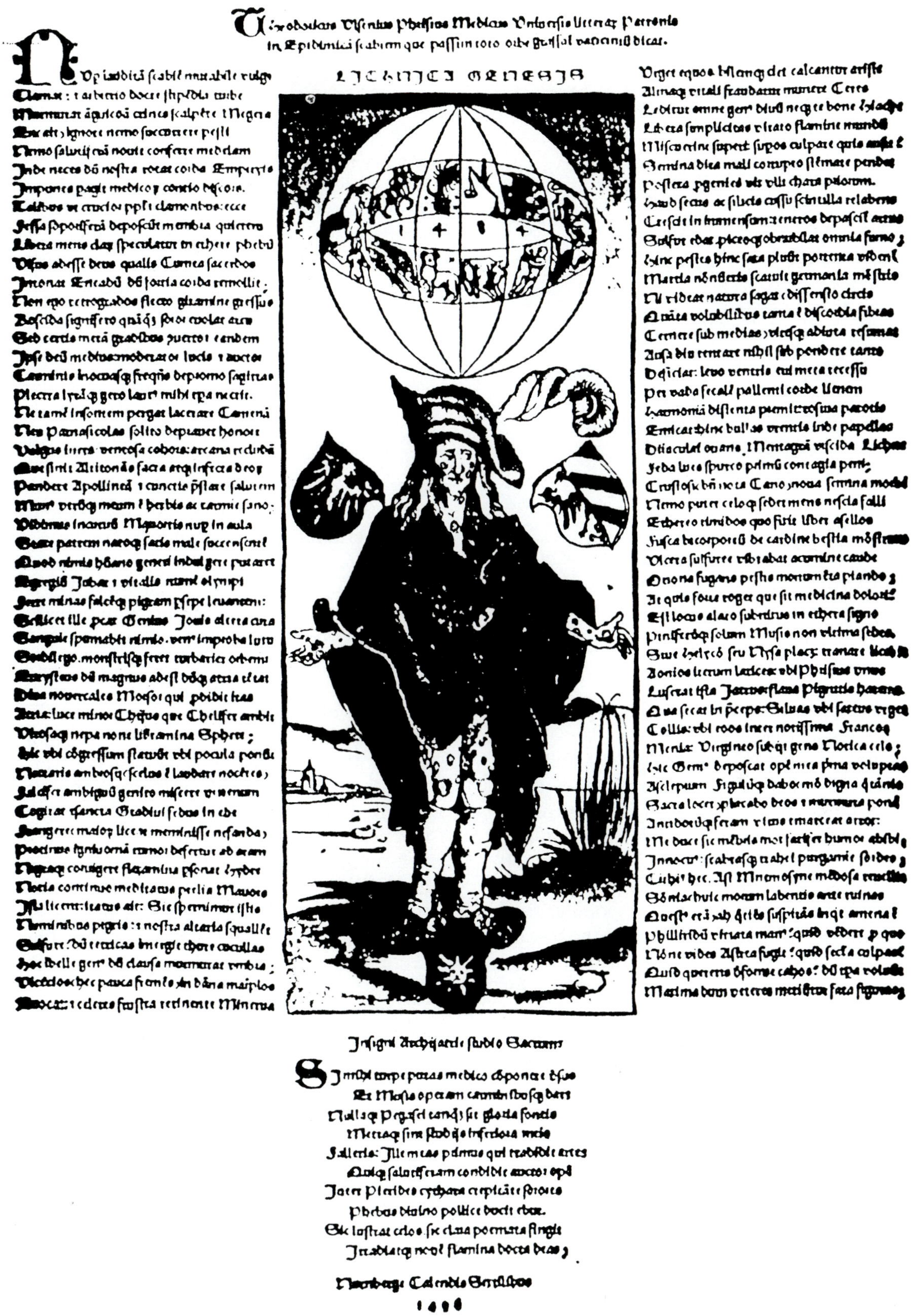

Figure 1. First Illustration of a Syphilitic Patient. A leaflet written by Theodorico Ulcenio, a physician from Nuremberg, demonstrating the astrological origin of morbus gallicus, the conjunction of Saturn and Jupiter. The illustration is by Albert Durer, 1496.

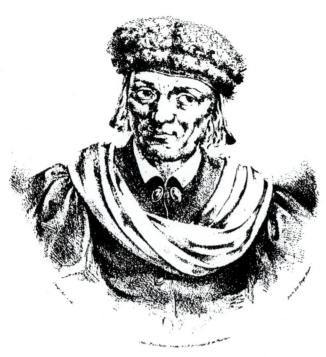

Figure 2. *Nicolo Leoniceno. A famous Italian physician who published the first treatise* (Libellus de epidemia, quam vulgo morbum gallicum vocant, 1497) *in which he asserted that the disease is very old and was already known by Hippocrates and Galen.*

didn't become popular until 1717, thanks to a work by Daniel Turner titled *Syphilis*.

Grünpeck first studied for the priesthood and was ordained; later, he obtained a degree in medicine. In the latter field he earned a good deal of prestige. In addition, he was secretary to Emperor Maximilian I.

Though it was popularly believed that the French disease was contracted through sexual intercourse, Grünpeck, under the sway of astrology, a popular field of study at the time, stated in his work that the disease was caused by the influence of the conjunction of the sun and a number of planets. He was to pay dearly for his credulity, along with his skeptical attitude toward the possibility of sexual transmission: he, like other members of the clergy, came down with syphilis. After suffering for three years with the illness, he described in great detail both the characteristics and evolution of his cutaneous lesions. In a later work, *Libellus . . . de mentulagra morbo rabido et incognito* (*Small Book . . . on the Fierce and Unknown Mentulagra disease*), he used the word *mentulagra*, a word derived from the Latin *mentula*, or virile member, to describe what he had previously called the French disease. The title demonstrates that, in the end, Grünpeck came to see the relationship between the Gallic disease, the male member, and sexual relations.

After the publication of Grünpeck's study, a number of other writers, especially those from Italy, published works on *morbo gallico*, including Bartolomeo Steber,[13] Nicolás Leoniceno,[1] Johannes Widman,[14] Antonio Benivieni,[15] and many others[16, 17] (Fig. 2).

THE FIRST WORKS FROM SPAIN

Only later did the theory of the American origin of syphilis come into being. According to this argument, it was Columbus' men who contracted the disease on the first or second voyage and then introduced it into Europe. The theory may be groundless and, for that very reason, early works on the subject written by Spanish authors merit discussion.

The first Spanish author to write about *morbo gallico* was a bishop and a physician from Valencia, Gaspar Torella,[18] who was also a relative of Rodrigo Borgia, the man who, as Alexander VI, sat on the throne of St. Peter in Rome. In view of the alarming spread of the French disease, the pope charged Torella with treating those affected, both within and beyond the Vatican walls. The fruit of his astute observations and fine clinical criteria is a work entitled *Tractatus cum consiliis contra pudendagram sive morbum gallicum* (*Treatise and Advice on the Pudendagra or Morbo Gallico*). Torella attempted to come up with a better name to replace *morbo gallico*; the result was *pudendagra*, from the Latin *pudendus*, or shameful, dishonest, disgraceful, a word used to refer to private parts of the human organism, also called the "shameful parts." This work was published in Rome in 1497. The author reports that in the Vatican alone he had treated seventeen patients suffering from the disease in only two months, a figure that reveals as much about the sexual activities of venerable members of the Vatican as it does about the contagious nature of the disease. In the appendix of the work, he includes a summary of clinical histories of five patients he treated. Subsequently, he published a number of additional works describing the pain and ulcerations brought on by *pudendagra* and other diseases.

Torella mentions that the illness appeared in Auvernia (a province of central France) and, from there, spread to other places, including Spain.

In 1498, Spanish physician Francisco López de Villalobos[2] published one of the most important works dealing with the subject, titled *Sumario de la medicina con Tratado sobre las Pestiferas Buvas* (*Summary of the Field of Medicine with a Treatise on the pestiferous Buboes*). Following a tradition popular at the time, even when dealing with scientific subjects, the author wrote his book in verse. López de Villalobos, an expert in clinical matters, described early symptoms and signs of the disease, as well as its evolution as manifested in the changing colors of lesions, the buboes, the gummata, the encordios, and even neurological problems caused by the disease in later stages. He sustained that the "sinful" disease was the fruit of licentious behavior. The fact that he describes lesions which would later be called "tertiary" reveals that during those early years the disease progressed rapidly in some patients, with a very short or no period of latency, evolving quickly to the tertiary phase.

López de Villalobos proposed the name "Egyptian scabies" as "it is a disease that existed in Egypt, which God visited upon the pharaoh in his 'nature' (that is, his procreative organ), as related in Genesis, chapter XI."

In 1500 in Rome, Spanish physician Pedro Pintor,[19] who at that time was already Alexander VI's physician, published a work titled *De morbo foetido et occulto bis temporibus affligente* (*Fetid and Hidden Disease Which, at the Same Time, Torments*). Pintor was widely famed in Rome and treated a growing number of syphilitics, both within and beyond the walls of the Vatican. Like his fellow countryman, he came up with a new name, *morbo foetido*, due to the repugnant odor of the ulcers. He stated that, prior to arriving in Rome, he had observed similar cases in Spain. He mentions something unheard of: the names and surnames of personages attached to the Roman court who suffered from the French disease.

Juan Almenar,[20] lord of Godella and Rocafort, originally from Valencia, published his work in Venice in 1502. It was titled *Libellus de morbo gallico, quem ita perfecte eradicare ostendit, ut numquam revertatur...* Due to its literary and scientific merit, the book came out in edition after edition and was translated into many languages. Almenar was the first to observe the ptyalism produced by mercury treatment; he recommended that it be administered in smaller doses and in conjunction with medicinal plants. In the face of the polemic surrounding the manner of contagion, he came up with a Solomonic solution: he stated that the sun, along with bad air, was the cause of the disease when contracted by priests, whereas in others it was due to kissing and sinful sexual relations.

In later years, news reached Spain that the natives of the islands of the West Indies (Caribbean), especially those living in present-day Haiti and the Dominican Republic, cured skin lesions with extracts from the bark of a tree called the *guayacán* (lignum vitae).

In 1517, Nicolás Poll,[21] an outstanding university professor and physician to Charles V, published a work entitled *De cura morbi gallici per lignum guayacanum libellus* (*Small Work on the Cure of the Gallic Disease with the Wood of the Guayacán*). A new edition appeared in Venice in 1535.

It was as a result of the curative properties, real or imagined, of the *guayacán*, or *guayaco*, that it was later named *palo santo*, or holy wood, and the sale of the wood, by decree of Charles V, became a monopoly of the Plugger brothers who had financed the monarch's ascension to the throne. They profited from the sale of the holy wood for many years and their fortune grew significantly as a result.

SYPHILIS: AN AMERICAN DISEASE?

Until 1526 it didn't occur to anyone, either in Spain or any other European country, to suspect, much less assert, that the French disease had come from America. In that year, Gonzalo Fernández de Oviedo[22] published a work titled *De la Natural Historia de las Indias*, better known as the *Sumario*. In this history, he describes a number of medicinal plants found in the New World, and in the chapter on lignum vitae, he says, "The principal virtue of this wood is its ability to cure buboes (thus did he refer to the disease which, in Spain, was better known as *bubas*) . . . that disease that came from the indies, and is very common among the indians, but is not as dangerous in those parts as in these, since the Indians of the islands cure themselves easily with this wood."

The same author, in 1535, published his *Historia general y natural de las Indias, islas y tierra firme del mar océano* (*General and Natural History of the Indies, Islands and Mainland of the Ocean Sea*). In this work, Fernández de Oviedo once again insists that buboes originated in America, and adds, "Many times, when in Italy, I laughed when I heard the Italians talking about the *French* disease and the French calling it the *Neapolitan* disease; when in truth, they would have been correct in calling it the *Indian disease*. And that this is true will be understood in this chapter and due to the vast experience with holy wood and *lignum vitae*, with which this terrible disease of buboes, more than with any other medicine, is cured, because so great is divine forgiveness that wherever possible, He, in His mercy, provides the remedies to heal our guilt, our trials, our sins, wherever these are found."

Was it this ancient maxim, that "Wherever God sends punishment or disease, there He also sends the cure," that led Fernández de Oviedo to claim that syphilis was American in origin?

But who is this individual who so arrogantly laughed at Italians and French and countless physicians, many of them highly respected, who spoke and wrote about the Gallic disease? What value have the opinions and affirmations of a layman who, long after they have published their works, decides to contradict the most learned physicians and surgeons of all Europe?

The future "Chronicler of the Indies" was, for a time, a page at the royal court. Later he was a scribe in Madrid. Finally, he found a job as inspector in the gold mines of Darien (present-day Colombia).

In that capacity, he traveled to the West Indies, twenty years after the outbreak of the first major syphilis epidemic, and approximately ten years after the introduction of the first black African slaves into the islands of the Caribbean.

In the first place, though he mentions that many Indians suffer from buboes, nowhere in his history does he suggest that he has actually seen anyone with the disease, nor does he attempt to describe these buboes. And, in the second place, the treponematosis most widely spread through the known world, prior to Columbus' voyage, was yaws which, in the Caribbean, was called *pián*. As black Africans suffered from yaws, and the matter has yet to be sufficiently studied, it is impossible to state whether they introduced the disease into America, as was the case with malaria and yellow fever, or if yaws was already there, having been introduced by the first human beings in the New World who migrated through the Bering Strait—at the time a land bridge—and from there spread throughout North and South America in the course of several thousand years.

Yaws is a skin disease found in tropical areas, one which affects children in particular. Its course is benign. The information that leads Fernández de Oviedo to conclude that what he called buboes was present in American was more likely a reference to yaws rather than syphilis.

Fernández de Oviedo asserts that the Spanish who accompanied Columbus on his voyages were responsible for taking buboes to Spain, and that from there it spread to Italy and eventually the rest of Europe.

Twenty or thirty years after the publication of the first works on the Gallic disease, the majority had been forgotten, as most of those editions were very small and available to very few.

The history of Fernández de Oviedo marks the beginning of a new period in historical interpretations based on his erroneous affirmations. Because he was an eye witness and lived for twenty years in the New World, his words carried added weight and were subsequently cited as articles of faith by authors who were at times less than scrupulous in checking their facts.

This is true of other early works on the history of the Americas, such as those by Fray Ramón Pané,[24] Fray Bartolomé de las Casas,[25] Pedro Martir de Anglería,[26] and Pedro Cieza de León.[27] These writers, basing their statements at times on their own observations and at times on references made by other, the latter being the case of Anglería, mention buboes as a disease carried by the aboriginal population. They describe a skin disease that temporarily disfigures the face, or they mention it in conjunction with descriptions of medicinal plants, like the sarsaparilla, used by the native in the treatment of skin diseases. The single individual who not only saw persons affected by the disease but also came down with buboes was the young Italian Girolamo Benzoni,[28] but that happened almost 80 years after the outbreak of the syphilis epidemic in Naples and, in any event, his illness was not syphilis. The categorical affirmations of Fernández de Oviedo and, possibly, corroborating statements by the other chroniclers mentioned above, became the evidence physicians used, beginning in 1525, to pronounce America the cradle of the French disease.

Among these physicians is Ruy Díaz de Isla[29] who, in 1539, published his *Tratado sobre el mal serpentino que vulgarmente en España se llama buvas...* (*Treatise on the Serpentine Disease, Popularly Known as Buboes in Spain...*). The author was a respectable 77 years of age when he published the book, and perhaps due to the natural deterioration of his memory, the work contains serious historical errors and lies which invalidate much of its contents. His work was forgotten until, in the 18th century, Jean Astruc,[30] in his bibliographic searches, came across it and made it the incontrovertible basis for his assertion that syphilis came from America.

Among other errors and fallacies, the author states that "Finding himself in Barcelona (in reference to the arrival of Columbus, in March 1493), he offered his services to *numerous* sailors attacked by this disease, who were on board the same ship commanded by Christopher Columbus." Columbus did not sail to Barcelona; he went by land. He was not accompanied by numerous sailors, but rather by a handful of officers and seven Indians. And not one of them suffered from any disease, much less one causing the very visible lesions that accompany syphilis. In addition, he affirms that he has been treating patients suffering from the "serpentine disease" for more than 40 years, which would indicate that he was seeing syphilitics even before Columbus' first voyage and, of course, before the outbreak of the syphilis epidemic in Naples.

It is curious that now, when all of Europe is talking of the French disease, this physician from the All Saints Hospital of Lisbon decides to propose a new name, the serpentine disease.

Another physician frequently cited by authors beginning in the seventeenth century is Nocolás Monardes,[31] who, in 1565, published *De las cosas que nos yienen de nuestras Indias occidentales y que sirven para el arte de curar* (*On the Things that Come From Our West Indies and that Serve the Curative Arts*). The work of this physician from Seville has true merit, except when he wanders into the realms of fantasy and myth, inspired by certain travelers and correspondents.

Monardes was dedicated to collecting information about the uses and properties of medicinal plants brought back by Spaniards who had traveled to the New World, especially those who had been to the Caribbean and, later, to New Spain (present-day Mexico) and South America. He experimented with the plants he received and thus became the first clinical pharmacologist of the Renaissance.

As for syphilis, he did not, unfortunately, question the historical accuracy of Fernández de Oviedo's account, but instead accepted and repeated it, almost word for word. In effect, he wrote, "Buboes came from the Indies. Perhaps it was Lord, Who sent the buboes disease, Who also provided the remedy. Because buboes came from the Indies, the first cases from Santo Domingo. Buboes are common among the Indians, and familiar to them, just as small pox is among us, and almost all the Indians, men and women, have them, since among them it is widespread, and the disease came in this way."

THE 400-YEAR-OLD CONTROVERSY

The works of the chroniclers of the Indies mentioned above, especially those of Pané, Fernández de Oviedo, and the physicians Ruy Díaz de Isla and Monardes, became the "solid bases" for theories of the American origin of syphilis. As a result, there arose a controversy between those who accepted the gratuitous affirmations of Fernández de Oviedo and those who maintained that syphilis did not originate in America but, rather, was a disease that had long existed in the Old World.

In a recently published work, Crosby[32] asks, "Where did syphilis come from? If the answer is America, we can be almost certain that it happened in 1493 or shortly after." He goes on to say that "In 1513 he (Fernández de Oviedo) traveled to the Indies where he spent most of the remainder of his life. No one can doubt that he had plenty of opportunity to learn as much as possible about the alleged American origin of this disease." Finally, he adds, "The third well-known member of this school of thought was a physician, Ruy Díaz de Isla, who, in a book published for the first time in 1539, maintains that he treated some of Columbus' men who had contracted syphilis in America in 1492 and that he observed the rapid spread of the disease in Barcelona." After offering this information, he concludes, without much conviction, that syphilis probably did originate in America. Nevertheless, it is important to remember that Fernández de Oviedo did not come to America in order to do research about anything, much less to investigate the French disease, and that his reference to the illness is circumstantial and bereft of historical context.

No one denies that an epidemic of syphilis began in Naples in March and April of 1495, or that the disease was carried to France by members of Charles VIII's army who had been infected in Italy, or that, on returning to their countries of origin, they spread the disease, and syphilis thus turned into a pandemic, the worst pandemic of syphilis experienced to date.

The problem lies in establishing, without a shadow of a doubt, whether it was that small group of men who accompanied Columbus on his return from his first and second voyages, who came back from America carrying the disease.

The first conundrum, for which there can be no satisfactory explanation, is as follows: Columbus returned from the West Indies at the beginning of 1493; that is, he arrived at Puerto de Palos on March 15 of that year. The epidemic began, as we have stated several times, during March and April of 1495, in other words, two years after his return.

A part of the fleet that made the second voyage returned to Spain in February 1494. Of the 1,500 men on this voyage, with few exceptions the only returnees were the crew members of the twelve small ships that made up the fleet. These men arrived somewhat more than a year before the epidemic broke out in Naples.

Had the Spaniards who went with Columbus on his first and second voyages returned infected with syphilis, it seems logical that the disease would have broken out in the Spanish cities of Puerto de Palos and Seville, in the region of Andalucia, to which they returned, and that it would have broken out with a virulence similar to that with which it manifested itself later in Naples. And from those cities, it would then have spread to the rest of Spain. But history reports nothing of the kind.

Table I is a brief chronological summary of the most important dates related to Columbus' first voyages and the syphilis epidemic. As the information in the table makes clear, there is no cause and effect relationship between said voyages and the outbreak of syphilis in Naples.

The second point to be discussed is the physical condition of the Spaniards and Indians who arrived in Spain. As for the second, Columbus, in his diary,[33] relates the following: "This people should be very useful and of lively intelligence, as I have observed that they learn quickly all that is said to them. . . . All have wide foreheads, wider than those of any other peoples I have seen to date. They have large and beautiful eyes. . . . In general, they have no fat on their bellies but, rather, graceful figures. All were as naked as the day their mothers brought them into this world, even the women, though I saw only one very young woman. All were of good build and had beautiful bodies. All I saw were young, not one of them being more than thirty years old."

The Indians Columbus presented to the king and queen of Spain were wearing only a loin cloth and thus their physical beauty was on display, as well as the fact that not one suffered a skin lesion that might be attributed to syphilis. The Spanish crew members who returned were likewise free of lesions that could be attributed to the disease.

It is true that the captain of the Pinta, Martín Alonso Pinzón, returned ill and died a few weeks later, but it was of a "common illness," not the disease that first appeared two years later in Italy. What's more, had the

TABLE I

Chronological Summary: Columbus' Early Voyages and the Outbreak of Syphilis in Europe

Date	Columbian Chronology:	Chronology of an Epidemic
	1492	
August 3	Columbus leaves from the port of Palos de Noguer to explore a new route to the Indies.	
October 12	He arrives at the Island of Guanahani, which he names El Salvador.	
	1493	
January 9	Columbus and 44 men depart from the Island of Hispaniola (today, Haiti and the Dominican Republic) for Spain.	
March 15	After a difficult and dangerous crossing, Columbus arrives at the port of Palos and sends an urgent message to the king and queen of Spain, who are in Barcelona.	
April 10	At the king's behest, Columbus leaves Seville, accompanied by a few officers and seven American Indians. The party is greeted enthusiastically by people in the towns of southern Spain.	
16	Columbus enters Barcelona in triumph. He is received by the king, the queen, members of the court, and a crowd of onlookers.	
30	Columbus returns to Seville to prepare for his second voyage.	
September 25	Second voyage begins, with a fleet of 17 ships and more than 1,500 men.	No cases of the venereal disease that will later be known as syphilis reported in Spain.
December	Columbus arrives at Hispaniola. A severe epidemic of flu or measles breaks out among the Spaniards and is spread to the native population, resulting in a high mortality rate among the latter.	
	1494	
February	Twelve of the seventeen ships begin the return to Spain, each with only the necessary crew members.	
April 15	The expeditionary fleet arrives.	Spaniards and Indians arriving in Spain on both voyages are in good health, showing no evidence of skin lesions.

TABLE I

Chronological Summary: Columbus' Early Voyages and the Outbreak of Syphilis in Europe

Date	Columbian Chronology:	Chronology of an Epidemic
	FRENCH INVASION OF ITALY	
Summer	On orders from Charles VIII, King of France, a large army, including regular French troops and mercenaries from France, Germany, Poland, Austria, Switzerland, and other countries, is organized.	
Autumn	The army, consisting of more than 30,000 men, leaves from Lyon, France, for Italy.	
October	Charles and his troops cross the Alps and advance rapidly into the region of Milan.	According to Leoniceno, the first cases of venereal disease appear around this time in Naples. The disease will later be called *morbus napolitanus*.
December 31	Charles enters Rome in triumph. A grand parade is organized. The pope takes refuge in the Castle of Saint Angel.	
	1495	
January 31	The Pope and Charles negotiate an agreement according to which the latter will respect the integrity of the Papal States if the former will encourage the king of Naples to resign. The army leaves Rome, enroute for Naples.	
February 22	Another triumphal entry, this time into Naples. Soldiers turn to pillage, theft, and rape.	
March and April		Many soldiers fall victim to venereal disease and fever. *Morbus napolitanus* becomes a violent epidemic.
May 20	For strategic reasons, and because so many of his soldiers are sick, Charles VIII begins his retreat.	
July 6	Battle of Fornobo (the only battle produced in the course of the invasion). Italian troops routed.	Italian soldiers reportedly infected with *morbus napolitanus*.
October	Army reaches France where the troops are demobilized. Mercenaries return to countries of origin.	Epidemic of venereal disease in Lyon, Paris, and other French cities. The disease is called *morbus gallicus*. It spreads to Germany, Poland, Flanders, Austria, and the rest of Europe. According to Torella, the disease travels from Auvernia, France to Spain, where it is called St. Clement's disease.

TABLE I

Chronological Summary: Columbus' Early Voyages and the Outbreak of Syphilis in Europe

Date	Columbian Chronology:	Chronology of an Epidemic
	1496	
April 22	Parliament in Paris passes an edict to prevent the spread of the disease.	
		During 1496, *morbus gallicus* spreads to Hungary, the Balkans, Russia, Greece, and, in the following years, to India, China, and Japan.
Final months of 1496		Publication of the first papers on *morbus gallicus*.

disease been syphilis, he should have infected at least his wife, and the same would have been true for other crew members.

As for the second voyage, Hernández-Morejón,[34] commenting on the lack of logic and factual data to support an argument for the American origin of syphilis, states that "Diego Alvarez de Chanca was the physician who, on the king's orders, accompanied Christopher Columbus on his second voyage. He describes with extraordinary care and a wealth of detail that is almost annoying, the events of the trip and the customs of the aborigines, as well as the illnesses of the members of the Spanish expedition. Can one possibly believe that a physician who reports so scrupulously on matters that have nothing to do with his field would have forgotten to mention an illness whose cutaneous manifestations are evident to even the most superficial of observers? This is even more inconceivable given that he does describe all the other illnesses that afflicted members of the crew during the crossing."

The third problem that requires explanation is why Spanish physicians like López de Villalobos who, beginning in 1497, were publishing works on syphilis, never so much as mention the hypothesis which holds that the disease originated in America. All of these early authors, during the three decades subsequent to the outbreak in Naples, give the disease various names and refer to a variety of possibilities, such as Egypt and, later and more concretely, France, as the site of the disease's origin.

How are we to explain, then, that a layman, a former mine inspector, a self-appointed historian (for which he must be given credit) comes up with the key to the mystery, affirming, as he does, that syphilis originated in America? How credible is such an affirmation, overlooking, as it does, studies and research findings by dozens of physicians, some of them very learned, not one of whom ever entertained a thought of said origin?

Another important point must be considered in re-

lation to the Spaniards in the New World. The chronicles and histories of America were begun one or two decades after Columbus's first voyage. The authors of these works mention that some Spaniards contracted buboes–almost certainly pián–an illness that, all agree, developed in benign fashion. If, in Europe, syphilis affected its victims with such virulence, the same should have happened to the Spaniards in America. However, nowhere in the histories or chronicles of this period is any event of the kind noted.

What is more, the social structure of peoples in the Americas did not create conditions favorable for the development of prostitution and the diseases associated with that practice. Leaders or chiefs could have as many wives as they wished; the rest of the population married early. All shared the fruits of agriculture, fishing, and other activities providing sustenance to members of each culture; no one was obliged to prostitute herself as a result of want.

In Europe, several decades after the outbreak of syphilis in Naples, physicians began to describe cases of inherited syphilis. In America, the chroniclers or historians provide extremely precise information on epidemics such as small pox, measles, and others that were brought from the Old World to the New. However, neither these writers nor physicians who arrived later in America mention a single case of inherited syphilis, with the exception of those cases that originated in Europe and were brought to America.

As the theory of the American origin of syphilis is based almost exclusively on historical references, we have limited this discussion to that aspect of the debate. Nevertheless, it is clear that a broader, more complete study must take into account other facets of this issue, including the biological, ethnological, genetic, and immunological. For example, a study on the origin of spirochetes of the genus *Treponema* which, according to Cockburn[35] and Hackett,[36] come from tropical Africa, has aroused tremendous interest.

In conclusion, we have an irrefutable historical fact, that of a violent outbreak of syphilis in Naples in 1495, a phenomenon which coincided with the presence of an invading force consisting of more than 30,000 soldiers led by French King Charles VIII. The invasion took place two years after Columbus returned from his first voyage and one year after he and a portion of his crew members turned from the second voyage. Further, we know that when members of Charles' army returned to France or, in the case of the mercenaries, to their countries of origin; these soldiers spread the disease throughout Italy and a good part of the rest of Europe.

In Naples there arose epidemiological conditions appropriate to the transformation into a violent epidemic of a disease that heretofore seems to have been benign in character and sporadic in appearance.

In view of the above, it is evident that the theory of the American origins of syphilis may be based on historical errors that have been repeated by authors past and present, as though these errors were proven facts.

ACKNOWLEDGMENT

This article was translated by Mary Ellen Fieweger.

REFERENCES

1. Leoniceno N. Libellus de Epidemia quam vulgo morbum gallicum vocant. Venecia. Aldus Manutius Romanus, June, 1497.
2. López de Villalobos F. El Sumario de la Medicina, con un tratado sobre las pertíferas buvas. Madrid: Impta. de I. Cosano, 1948 (First edition, 1498).
3. Di Vigo G. Práctica in arte chirurgica copiosa. Roma: 1514.
4. Cicerón M. T. De finibus honorum et malorum. De invensione. Roma, 45 B.C.
5. Horacio FQ. Horatii Flacci Opera. Parmae: Typis Bodonianus, 1789.
6. Ovidio P. Ars amandi.—Amores, 4a elegía. Roma: 8 A.D.
7. Lewinshon R. Storia dei Costumi Sessuali. Milano: Sugar Editore. 1963.
8. Abraham IJ. The Early History of Syphilis. Brit. J. Surg. 32:15, 1944.
9. Cumanus M. Pustulitis. Navaro: 1495.
10. Holcomb RC. The Antiquity of Syphilis. Medica Life XLII. New York: No. 172–183 of New Series, 1935.
11. Allen-Pusey WM. The History and Epidemiology of Syphilis. Springfield Ill: Ch. Thomas, 1933.
12. Grünpeck J. Tractatus origene de pestilentiale Scorra sive mala de Franzos, Ausburg: 1496.
13. Steber B. De morbus gallicus. Venecia: 1497–98.
14. Widmann I. De pustulis quae vulgata nomine dicuntur mal de Franzos. Rome: 1497.
15. Benivieni A. De abditis non nullis ae mirandis morborum et sanatiorum causis. Venecia: 1500.
16. Sudholf K. Der Ursprung der Syphilis. Leipzig: Vogel, 1913.
17. Jeanselme AB. Histoire de la syphilis, son origin, son expansion. París: Doin, 1931.
18. Torella G. Tractatus cum consilii contra pudendagram sive morbum gallicum. Rome: 1497.
19. Pintor P. De morbo foetido et occulto his temporibus affligente. Rome: 1500.
20. Almenar J. Libellus de morbo gallico, quem ita perfecte iradicare ipsum ostendit, ut numquam revertatur. Venecia: 1502.
21. Poll N. De cura morbi gallici per lignum guayacanum libellus (1517). Venecia: 1535 (Colección Basilia, 1536).
22. Fernández de Oviedo G. De la Natural Historia de las Indias. Ramón de Petras. Toledo: 1526.
23. Fernández de Oviedo G. Historia general y natural de las Indias (5 vol.). Gráficas orbe, Madrid: 1959. (La 1a. edición fue de 1535).
24. Pané R. Fray Treatise of Friar Ramon on the Anitiquities of the Indians. . . . En: Columbus, Ramon Pané and the Beginnings of American Anthropology, por E.G. Bourne, Proc. Amer. Antiquit. Soc. Worcester: 1906.
25. Casas B. de las Historia de las Indias. (3 vol.). Pondo de Cult. Económica México: 1951.
26. Angleria PM. de Fuentes históricas sobre Colón y América. Impta. San Fco. de Sales. Madrid: 1892.
27. Cieza de León P. La Crónica del Perú. Espasa-Calpe. Madrid: 1962.
28. Benzoni G. Historia del Mondo Nuovo. Edic. facsimilar (1572) Graz (Austria): A Kadem. Druck V. VEslang: 1969.
29. Díaz de Isla R. Tractado llamado fructo de todos los Sanctos: contra el Mal Serpentino venido de la Isla Española. . . . Sevilla: Andrés de Burgos, 1542.
30. Astruc J. De morbis venereis. Libri novem inquibus disseritur-tum de origine. G. Cavalier. Lutetiae Parisoirum: 1740.
31. Monardes W. De las cosas que nos vienen de nuestras Indias Occidentales y que sirven para el arte de curar. Sevilla: 1580.
32. Crosby AW. El intercambio transoceánico. Consecuencias biológicas y culturales a partir de 1492. Univ. Autón. de México. México: 1991.
33. Colombo C. II Giornale di bordo di Cristoforo Colombo. Schwarz editore. Milán: 1960.
34. Hernández-Morejón A. Historia Bibliográfica de la Medicina Española (7 Vol.). Impta. Vda. De Jordán. Madrid: 1842.
35. Cockburn TA. The origen of the Treponematosis. Bull. World Health Org. 24:221, 1961.
36. Hackett CJ. On the Origin of the Human Treponematoses. Bull. World Health Org. 29:7–41, 1963.

Chapter 7

Genetic Difference Between Europeans and Indians: Tissue and Blood Types

Clara Gorodezky, D.Sc., Ph.D

ABSTRACT

When Columbus reached America, the continent probably was inhabited by 15 to 30 million natives. Today Mexico has 68 different Indian tribes based on a linguistic classification; 5 million people speaking different languages are registered. However, 95% of the Mexican population are Mestizos who represent a triracial genetic admixture: Caucasian genes from the Spanish conquerors, an Oriental gene-pool derived from the native Indians, and a small contribution of black genes from the African slaves brought by the Spaniards to America. The admixture started around 1500, and it is now very difficult to distinguish phenotypically one group from another; and the Mestizos from the Indians. Therefore, proteins with multiple inherited alternate forms like the major histocompatibility complex (in humans the HLA proteins, also called HLA antigens) and several blood markers are valuable tools and crucial elements to trace human migrations, to define degree of admixture, and to explore the impact of genetics on the epidemiology of the different populations. The distribution of blood group system markers throughout western Europe is very uniform. In contrast, there are two alternative protein forms that are almost never seen in Mongolians as compared with European Caucasians. Although distinctive blood group markers also exist in Orientals, several groups have a very distinctive pattern, such as the Senoi from Malay, the Tharons from Burma, and the Ainu from Japan. We analyzed four Mexican Indian tribes and, as in Amerindians, blood group O is extremely high; several other blood groups are increased in the same way as they are in Mongolians, Orientals, and Amerindians. Other proteins may be present in high frequency because they may protect against diseases or other conditions present in the environment in which a tribal group has lived. Certain Rh genes (such as R_2) are present probably because they confer selective advantage to these groups. The genes of the HLA complex control molecules (class I and class II antigens) that function as recognition elements of foreign proteins or of proteins present in an individual (foreign and self antigens). Thus, an immune response against infectious agents or foreign proteins occurs only when the immune system is exposed to them in combination with an HLA antigen. HLA genes also are involved in disease resistance and susceptibility to many autoimmune diseases and to certain infections, such as leprosy or tuberculosis. Because of the extraordinary variety in their forms, the HLA genes are markers of individuality and are of great help in population genetics, anthropology, and in analyzing diseases with a genetic background. We studied five different Indian groups (Nahuas, Tarahumaras, Mazahuas, Mixtecos, and Lacandones) and Mestizos. The genetic pattern of the Indians is very restricted, and certain antigens seem to be found nearly exclusively in Indians. The Mestizos are clearly a triracial group;

Department of Immunogenetics, INDRE, SSA

and the Lacandones, who belong to the Mayan family, are the most homogeneous tribe. DR4 is remarkably high in them, suggesting either that it protects them from harmful environmental factors (selective advantage) or that the high frequency in early ancestors was increased by inbreeding. The genetic similarities demonstrate that the Nahuas and Tarahumaras are closely related and the Lacandones and Mixtecos, although belonging to different families, had a common origin. The ancient ancestors of Mexican Indians are Japanese, Koreans, Chinese, Thais, and Malays, as shown by the genetic similarities. Disease-association studies in Indians indicate that ankylosing spondylitis depends strongly on the presence of B27, and populations with a low frequency of B27 have a low prevalence of the disease. Pima Indians do not suffer with type I diabetes (insulin-dependent diabetes mellitus [IDDM]), but non-IDDM is a common disease among them. It is now evident that certain HLA class II genes play an important role in the expression of IDDM. Hepatic cirrhosis is frequent in Mazahuas but not in others; we suggest that a Caucasian gene (HLA-B8) that remained after an important admixture, is partially responsible for the disease. These are all examples of how isolated populations provide fertile ground for studying diseases and migration patterns, and how the admixture has given rise to new ethnic groups where the genetics and environment have jointly acted to define the features of the peoples in the New World.

W
hen Columbus and the early Spanish explorers asked the natives where they came from, they recited long histories of tribal migrations, and showed them gigantic bones. Most of the Spanish chroniclers realized, however, that these bones did not belong to natives' ancestors[1] because they had some idea of the ancient existence of huge animals like the mammoths.

The original Americans are now believed to have originated in the Eastern Hemisphere. Man came to this continent as a hunter following herds of animals through the Bering Straits. Weapons discovered, many times in association with extinct animal bones, at more than 200 sites establish human habitation on the North American continent for a period of 30,000 to 40,000 years.[1] When Columbus sighted land in 1492, America had a total of 13 to 15 million Indians. In Mexico alone, 5000 archeological sites and innumerable remains exist, suggesting that the number of Indians probably equaled those in South America.[2]

The first inhabitants of Mexico were primitive hunters who traveled in small groups until the herds of animals disappeared. This forced people to establish relatively permanent settlements, probably between 300 to 1500 BC. The descendants of those early people still have many of the physical/anthropological characteristics of Orientals.

Today Mexico has 68 different Indian tribes classified from a linguistic viewpoint. According to the 1980 census, Mexico has 5 million people speaking various Indian languages. These data are, however, an underestimation,

because children under 5 years of age were not considered.[4] The Indians belong to five large linguistic groups that span at least 50 centuries: Tarasco, Macromaya, Maromixteco, Macronahua, and Macroyuma.[3] These groups are distributed among 12 families.[4]

Besides these peoples, Mexico is mainly composed of Mestizos (constituting 95% of the actual population) who represent a triracial admixture of Caucasian genes of Spaniard origin, an Oriental gene pool from the Indians, and a small amount of black genes from the slaves brought by the Spaniards mainly from Senegal, Morocco, and the Gold Coast. (At the end of the 17th Century these slaves were Bantus from the Congo River.) The admixture with the Spaniards started around 1521, when the different Indian groups intermixed with their conquerors. By 1640, about 150,000 black slaves were in Mexico, living mainly along the coasts and adding to the genetic mix that gave rise to the Mestizos.[5]

It is often difficult to distinguish the Mestizos from the Indians. The mother language may be a helpful marker but genetic identity cannot be assured even though many tribes have preserved their unique cultural and linguistic features. Because protein synthesis is directed by the genes, naturally-occurring protein complexes with multiple inherited alternate forms (polymorphic systems) such as the HLA complex and some blood factors are remarkable tools for showing genetic differences and similarities between populations. The analysis of population genetics using these protein markers as a tool is a fascinating topic, because through them the biological and epidemiological impact of human invasions and migrations on the genetic structure of today's Mexican Indians can be unraveled.[6,7]

This article analyzes the genetic composition of the Mexican Indians and demonstrates how it differs from the genetic patterns of Europeans. In addition, it shows how the HLA markers and blood group systems have influenced the health status and susceptibility to disease of the Mexican population.

DISTRIBUTION OF BLOOD GROUP SYSTEMS IN CAUCASIANS AND INDIANS

M
ost blood group systems are distributed uniformly among western European populations. The general pattern of the ABO system shows high gene frequencies of group O in the west (65 to 75%), of A in the middle (22 to 29%), and of B in the east (14 to 23%); A_2 is (in general) a typical European gene. This lack of diversity suggests that ABO groups respond more readily to natural selection resulting from variations in the environment than do most of the other red cell systems.[8,9]

In contrast, in the Eastern peoples, broadly described as Mongolians, from whom the North American Indians descend, groups A and B remain high, but the A_2 subgroup almost disappears. In another set of blood group antigens controlled by genes at a different locus, one form (the S allele) has an unexpectedly low frequency when compared with European Caucasians. The frequency of Rh negative individuals is also very low. Despite the great variety of ethnic groups living in Southeast and East Asia, genetic homogeneity also exists as a whole in this part of the globe. Certain aboriginal populations differ widely, such as the Senoi of Malaya, the Tharons of Burma (who are immigrants from China), and the Ainu of Japan, who are totally unique in their blood group frequencies compared with any other population in the world.[8,9]

We have analyzed blood group systems in four different Mexican Indian tribes (Lacandones, Tarahumaras, Mazahuas, and Mixtecos), and the main findings are shown in Table I. In addition to the Indians indicated here, about 44 other tribes have been studied and elegantly reviewed by Lisker.[10] It is clear that in general, group O of the ABO system is an Amerindian marker, although a certain degree of admixture with Caucasian and black genes is evident. Almost all are negative for K (Kell system) in contrast with Caucasians, and most of them have frequencies for one form of the P system (P1+) greater than 50%, as do other groups from Central and South America.[8,9,11] The high frequency of one Duffy antigen (Fy^a) is consistent with the values of other Amerindians, and similar numbers have been described only in Lapps, Chinese, Ainus, Koreans, and Asian natives.[8,9] The Diego Di^a antigen is undoubtedly a Mongoloid marker. Its distribution among Amerindians[10,11] is very variable but is absent in Caucasians, blacks, Polynesians, and Australian Aborigines.[8,9] The Xg^a locus shows frequencies above 50% in the Lancandones, similar to that in Caucasians and blacks; so this locus is not subject to natural selection forces, or its frequency is due to admixture. The distribution of one form of Kidd (Jk^a) varies, but its value is closer to Mongolians, as is the distribution of one form of Lewis antigen (Le^a). The gene frequencies of the Lutheran and Kp antigens show that geographical aspects might have influenced the variability found in these antigens in Indians, although in some of them white genes may have been fixed. Some contribution of black genes is observed in the MnSs systems, but the prevalence of the M and s genes is characteristic in Amerindians.[8-11]

The overall findings for the complex Rh-Hr system demonstrate that the distribution is similar to that of other Amerindians. However, certain genes are present at a high frequency in some groups; this is probably due to admixture, but perhaps because it confers some selective advantage in the particular environment those Indians inhabit.

Finally, it is important to mention that even if Indians have particular markers or frequencies, they are not "genetically pure," at least for blood group systems. This is clear from calculations of gene admixture. The data

---

TABLE I.

Similarities and Differences in Gene Frequencies of Blood Groups among Four Mexican Indian Tribes Compared with Other Populations

Blood Group System	Lacandon N=174	Tarahumara N=95	Mazahua N=100	Mixteco N=73	Mestizo N=295
ABO	U	U	U	U	U
Kell	O	N	C	N	O
P	C, B	C, B	B	C, B	C
Duffy	Between C & B Different from other tribes	Closest to O	Closest to O	Closest to O	C
Diego	U but like Tarahumara and Mestizos	close to Lacandon	O	O	close to Lacandon
Xg	C	O	(No data)	U	(No data)
Kidd	O	O	(No data)	O	(No data)
Lewis	U	U	U	U	B*
Lutheran	C	O	(No data)	U	C
Kp	U	U	(No data)	U	C, O, B
MnSs	O	U	U	U	C

*In distribution of polymorphic forms: U=Unique to Indians; N=no significant difference from any major racial group; C=like Caucasian; B=like Black; O=like Oriental; *=data incomplete.*

obtained for 36 different Mexican Indian tribes show that the Caucasian gene admixture ranges from 2.75% in Maya I to 33.1% in Mixteco I. Only Tzotzil, Huasteco, Huichol, and Seri show no admixture for the ABO system, although some degree of admixture is present for other systems.[10] The medical implications of these features will be further discussed.

THE HLA COMPLEX

An Example of Medical and Anthropological Transcendency

The HLA complex is of great interest because of the extent of its enormous polymorphism. Many genes are linked in the HLA complex forming particular combinations that probably contribute to protection against diseases that might have destroyed human populations.[12,13] The biological function of HLA molecules is to combine with the peptides of foreign antigens and to present them to receptors (T-cell receptors) on immune system cells (T-helper or T-cytotoxic cells) where they are recognized as foreign. This recognition system enables an individual to develop an immune response against the antigens and, therefore, to possess the capacity for protection against different diseases. The HLA is thus a regulation system of the T-cell mediated immune response.[14]

Another very important feature of the HLA genes is their participation in susceptibility and resistance to many diseases that are probably also influenced by other genes and factors. Today, more than 500 clinical entities are confirmed to be linked or associated with HLA genes. Among these are rheumatologic, allergic, autoimmune, neurologic, dermatologic, nephrologic, gastric, hepatic, hematologic, and some clearly infectious disorders.[15] Therefore, the HLA complex is an appropriate system to trace back diseases with a genetic background.

We have studied the HLA complex in five Indian tribes (Nahuas, Mazahuas, Tarahumaras, Mixtecos, and Lacandones) and several groups of Mestizos.[16–20] The frequencies between one group and another vary and show different degrees of admixture with Caucasian and black genes. It is evident that some genes are of higher frequencies in Indians, such as A2, A24, A31, B39, B35, B48, B51, B60, B61, Cw4, Cw7, DR2, DR4, DR8, DR12, DR14, and perhaps DQ7. Some of them are very close to Orientals and seem to be Indian markers (A31, Cw4, B35, B39, B48, DR4, DQ7). The Mestizos are clearly a triracial group with some antigenic frequencies that are closer to Caucasians, many others closer to Orientals, and very little contribution of black genes. The Lacandones, who belong to the Mayan family and live inside the jungle in the southeast of Mexico, are the most homogeneous group, with a very restricted pattern of HLA antigens and an extraordinarily high frequency of DR4, which, although it comes from Orientals, probably was established in this small population through inbreeding that gradually eliminated other alternative forms of DR. Alternatively, DR4 may be an immune response gene that conferred a selective advantage against infections.

The Lacandones are more genetically like the Mixtecos (who live in the state of Oaxaca, also southeast) than the other Indians. This means that the two tribes are ancestrally related and that they are genetically removed from the Uto-Aztecs, to whom the Nahuas and Tarahumaras belong. They are very close to the so-called Amerindians and to the Koreans and Japanese. The Oriental ancestral origin is evident. Comparing the HLA distribution with other Orientals, it is possible to trace migration routes and to distinguish several influences. The phylogenetic tree is composed of Japanese, Philippines, Malays, Koreans, Chinese, and Thais, therefore validating several migration waves at different times in the past. There are probably undemonstrated subtypes of B16, DR8, DR6, and DQ3 that may play an important role in the epidemiological status of the Indian groups.

IMPACT OF GENETIC PROFILE ON EPIDEMIOLOGY OF AMERINDIANS AND MESTIZO POPULATIONS

Amerindians contribute greatly to the understanding of HLA disease associations. These groups generally have good visual acuity and low frequencies of caries and otosclerosis. A good proportion of them have never been exposed to the tuberculosis or leprosy bacilli. However, they do have high antibody titers to different infectious agents. Among them are toxoplasma, trichinella, a wide variety of intestinal bacteria, and parasites. Local factors and contact with the Mestizo populations as well as with visitors of foreign origin have brought to them leishmaniasis, influenza infections, tuberculosis, onchocerciasis, and cysticercosis, diseases previously unknown among them.[7,10,11]

Similar unique disease patterns exist among the Indian tribes in South America. Three patterns of treponemal infection were observed among Yanomama and Makiritare in Brazil; the Cayapo show a high prevalence of spirochetal infection in the absence of clinical disease. Iodine deficiency without goiter was found in Yanomama. A new form of dwarfism was detected among the Yukpa in Venezuela. The irides of many Aymara Indians from Chile fail to dilate after the administration of drops of 1% mydracil, probably resulting from the presence of a double dose of a mutant gene on both chromosomes. Thirteen serotypically unique O strains of *Escherichia coli* have been found among the Yanomama, and the Mapuches from Chile have a higher proportion of oneriform psychoses than occurs among non-Indians (reviewed in Ref. 11).

ANKYLOSING SPONDYLITIS

Ankylosing spondylitis (AS) affects the sacroiliac and posterior intervertebral joints of the spine. The prevalence is high among Caucasians, intermediate among middle-Eastern groups, low in many Orientals, and absent from African blacks and Australian Aborigines. HLA-B27 is dramatically increased in ankylosing spondylitis patients, and the distribution of the antigen runs parallel with the geographical distribution of the disease. About 90% of the Caucasian patients are B27+ versus 4 to 13% in controls, and in Japanese patients 67 to 92% are B27+ versus only 0 to 2% in controls; among American blacks only 48% of the patients are B27 carriers compared with 2% of the controls.[22] In Mexican Mestizos, we found a frequency of 69% B27 positive patients and 5% among the controls.[23]

It is worthwhile to mention some examples among Amerindians. In tribes of the United States of America and Canada that have been studied (Haida, Bella Coola, and Pima), the frequency of B27 among the controls is high. In the Haida, where it is 51% in controls, a large proportion of the males (10%) have AS, and all of them are B27+ (100%). Among Bella Coola controls, 26% have been found to be B27 and again, 100% of the patients carry the antigen. In contrast, in the Pima population where the control frequency of B27 is 18%, 20% of randomly selected individuals had AS, but of these, only 57% were B27 positive. In the Mexican Indians we studied, the B27 frequency ranges from 0 in Lacandones to 2.5% in Mazahuas and 3.7% in Tarahumaras, and the disease seems to be rare or absent among them; only one Tarahumara had AS, and he was B27+. AS is clearly associated with HLA-B27 and probably is due, at least partly, to a Caucasian gene introduced in the Amerindian populations. By contrast, the Haida and Bella Coola from Western Canada possibly descend from Thais, Thai-Chinese, and Timors, who have a higher frequency of B27 than do the eastern Asia populations from which the Pima and Mexican Indians mainly descend. Thus, the B27 gene might have been present in especially high frequency in the small group of ancestors who founded the tribe and was fixed in these Indians through a "bottleneck" mechanism. When a population is derived from a small group that contained a limited number of alleles (alternative forms of a gene), the presence of those alleles is called the "founder effect." If this effect occurred in recent times, the population can be visualized as having passed through a "bottleneck": a period in which the population was drastically reduced in number, after which it expanded again.

DIABETES MELLITUS

Pima Indians do not suffer from insulin-dependent diabetes mellitus (IDDM); however, non-IDDM is common. It is familial and strongly related to obesity. Neel[24] suggested that the introduction of a steady food supply to people who have evolved a "thrifty genotype" leads to obesity, insulin resistance, and diabetes. The thrifty genotype involves the ability of insulin to maintain fat stores, despite resistance to glucose disposal. The Pimas adapted

successfully to desert life until this century, when increasing settlement of their area by people of European descent led to diversion of the tribe's water supply and disruption of their traditional agricultural way of life. Now the Pimas share many of the lifestyle habits of non-Indian Americans and are plagued by some chronic health problems that may be related to their changing history. Obesity and diabetes are two such problems.[25]

The gene responsible for non-IDDM is not HLA related. In contrast, IDDM depends greatly on some HLA class II genes. A clear association exists with DR3 and DR4 in all ethnic groups studied.[22] However, DNA analysis shows that the presence of one particular amino acid (aspartic acid) at position 57 of a class II HLA protein confers protection while another (arginine) at position 52 of another HLA protein leads to susceptibility.[26] Our findings in Mexican Mestizos[27] with IDDM show the contribution of DRB genes as well as those found in Japanese. Mexican Indians have low frequencies of the HLA antigens that are associated with IDDM, and the disease has not been detected in these groups. The data strongly support the hypothesis of diabetogenic genes located in the Class II region of the HLA complex.

HEPATIC CIRRHOSIS, RHEUMATOID ARTHRITIS, AND ALBINISM IN MEXICAN INDIANS

Alcohol consumption among Mexican Indians is usually high. The Mazahuas are used to drinking beer, which has about 6% alcohol, and 53% of the population are consumers. The Tarahumaras consume "tesguino", a corn spirit that is about 45% alcohol; and 74% are heavy consumers. The expectation is that the incidence of hepatic cirrhosis would be greater in Tarahumaras, but we found 7% prevalence of the disease among Mazahuas and not a single case in Tarahumaras. It has been shown that this disease is associated with an HLA Class I antigen, HLA-B8, in Caucasians[22]; not surprisingly, the frequency of B8 in Tarahumaras is 1.6% and in Mazahuas is 5.7%, even higher than in Mestizos (1.7%). Therefore, we suggested that the disease exists in Mazahuas because they have the HLA gene that predisposes to it, which must have been acquired from Caucasians because B8 is a Caucasian marker.[17] The Tarahumaras probably do not get the disease because, not having the susceptibility gene derived from Caucasians, they are genetically more protected.

Another example is rheumatoid arthritis. Tarahumaras do not seem to have a high prevalence of ankylosing spondylitis (AS), and the frequency of B27 is low (3.2%), but 17.8% have family antecedents of rheumatoid arthritis, and 7% have the disease; 72% (13/18 cases) have the class II HLA antigens that are associated with either adult or juvenile rheumatoid arthritis.[17] These data agree with many others supporting the theory that HLA genes are also susceptibility markers for diseases affecting the small joints.

Finally, albinism present in Lacandones due to inbreeding seems also to be HLA related. The three affected persons had the same series of Class I and Class II HLA proteins although they belonged to different families, and only 18.1% of the healthy sibs in the families (31/171) had these antigens ($p = <0.004$).

CONCLUSIONS

Isolated populations of the Americas provide a fertile ground for analysis of the mechanisms of HLA associations, for determining the effects of levels of HLA-linked genes on resistance or susceptibility to infections in these groups, and for studying the mechanisms of coevolution and selection that gave rise to the enormous variation in the HLA loci. What is the meaning of the great homogeneity of the genetic pattern in Amerindians? Have some HLA types been selected because they confer biological advantage against disease that can devastate human populations? Does the existence of an exceptionally large number of Amerindians who carry two different alternative forms of HLA protein indicate that there is a gene favoring this lack of homogeneity near the HLA genes? Is this an advantage to the species survival? All are questions that we hope will be answered in the near future by using the molecular approach to study more native groups and their diseases.

ACKNOWLEDGMENTS

Dr. Gorodezky is truly grateful to L. Castro, J. Flores, O. Hernandez, J.M. Carranza, G. de la Rosa, G. Cazares, J.A. Sierra, A. Martinez, G. Granados, V. Trejo, A. Olivo, R. Martinez, R. Martinez-Maranon, P.H. Caire, E. Torres, P.H. Lefevre-Witier, Instituto Nacional Indigenista; Instituto Nacional de Antropologia UNAM; and Fundacion Schweitzer for their very valuable help.

She is also grateful to the National Institutes of Health for financial support through contract NIH NO1-A1-62-S23.

The efforts of Jane Schultz, Ph.D., and Estelle Schwalb in revising Dr. Gorodezky's original paper are gratefully acknowledged.

REFERENCES

1. Peterson F. Earlyman in Mexico. Ch 1. In: Peterson F, ed, Ancient Mexico. An Introduction to the Pre-Hispanic Cultures, 2nd ed. New York: Capricorn Books, 1962, pp. 17–29.
2. Ramirez, Codice. Relación de los Indios que habitan esta Nueva España. México, 1944.
3. Swadesh M. Indian linguistic groups of Mexico. Escuela Nacional de Antropología e Historia. México, 1959.
4. Manrique CL, Demonte V, Garza Cuaron B, eds. Pasado y presente de las lenguas indígenas en México. In: Estudios lingüísticos de España y México. UNAM and Colegio de México A.C. 1990, pp. 387–420.
5. Chavero DA. Historia Antigua y de la Conquista. In: Riva-Palacio V, ed. Mexico a Través de los Siglos. 6th ed. Mexico: Editorial Cumbre S.A., 1967, pp. 741–763.
6. Kostyu D, Amos B. Mysteries of the Amerindians. Tissue Antigens 16:11, 1981.
7. Tsuji, K, Aizawa M, Sasasuki T. HLA 1991, Oxford, England; Oxford University Press, 1992.
8. Tills D, Kopec AC, Tills RE, eds. The Distribution of Human Blood Groups. Oxford: Oxford University Press, 1983.
9. Roychoudhury AK, Nei M, eds. Human Polymorphic Genes. World Distribution. New York: Oxford University Press, 1988.
10. Lisker R. Estudios realizados en grupos indigenas. In: Lisker R, ed. Estructura genética de la Población mexicana. México DF: Salvat Mexicana de Ediciones, S.A. 1981, pp. 41–96.
11. Salzano FM, Callegari-Jackes SM, eds. Discontinuous Genetic Variability: Description in South American Indians. A Case Study in Evolution. Oxford: Clarendon Press, 1988, pp. 138–162.
12. Bodmer JG, Marsh SGE, Albert ED, et al. Nomenclature for factors of the HLA system, 1990. Human Immunol 31:186–194, 1991.
13. Klein J. Of HLA, types, and selection: An essay on coevolution of MHC and parasites. Human Immunol 30:247–258, 1991.
14. Braciale TJ, Braciale VL. Antigen presentation: Structural themes and functional variations. Immunol Today 12:124–129, 1991.
15. Batchelor JR, McMichael AJ. Progress in understanding HLA and disease associations. Br Med Bull 43:156–183, 1987.
16. Gorodezky C, Castro-Escobar LE, Escobar-Gutierrez A. The HLA system in the prevalent Mexican Indian group: the Nahuas. Tissue Antigens 25:38–46, 1985.
17. Gorodezky C, Variación genética del MHC en la población mexicana, Histocmp Latamer 1:8–21, 1988.
18. Gorodezky C, Granados G, Flores J, et al. Genetic polymorphisms in Mixteco Indians from Mexico. Human Immunol 23:102. 1988.
19. De la Rosa G, Castro L, Flores J, et al. MHC profile of Lacandones: An isolated Mexican Maya tribe. Human Immunol 1990. 16th Annual ASHI Meeting, Los Angeles, p. 114.
20. Park MS, Gorodezky C, Terasaki P. HLA in a population of Mexicans In: Aizawa M. ed. HLA in Asia and Ocenia. Sapporo, Japan: Hokkaido University Press, 1986, pp. 291–294.
21. Baur MP, Neugebauer M, Deppe H, et al. Population analysis on the basis of deduced haplotypes from random families. In: Albert ED, Baur M, Mayr WR, eds. Histocompatibility Testing 1984, Berlin: Springer-Verlag, 1984, pp. 333–341.
22. Tiwari JL, Terasaki PI, eds. HLA and disease associations. New York: Springer-Verlag, 1985.
23. Fraga A, Gorodezky C, Lavalle C, et al. HLA-B27 in Mexican patients with ankylosing spondylitis. Arthritis Rheum 22:302–304, 1979.
24. Neel JV. The thrifty genotype revisited. In: The genetics of diabetes mellitus. Kobberling J, Tattersal RB, eds. Serono Symposium, London: Academic Press, 1982.
25. Knowler WC, Pettit DJ, Bennett PH, Williams RC. Diabetes mellitus in the Pima Indians: Genetic and evolutionary considerations. Am J Phys Anthropol 62:107–114, 1983.
26. Khalil I, d'Aauriol L, Gobet M, et al. A combination of HLA-DQB Asp57-negative and HLA-DQalpha Arg52 confers susceptibility to insulin-dependent diabetes mellitus. J Clin Invest 85:1315–1319, 1990.
27. Gorodezky C, Debaz H, Olivo A, et al. The contribution of HLA-DRB1, DQA1 and DQB1 genes for the susceptibility to type I diabetes (IDDM) in Mexicans. Tissue Antigens (submitted).

Chapter 8

Fauna, Flora, Fowl, and Fruit: Effects of the Columbian Exchange on the Allergic Response of New and Old World Inhabitants

John E. Salvaggio, M.D.

ABSTRACT

The Columbian Exchange has been described as "the most important event in human history since the end of the Ice Age." This interchange of many species of fauna, flora, fowl, and fruits resulted in new encounters between New and Old World inhabitants. Prominent among these were manifestations of allergic reactions to many of the new substances. Little imagination is required to reflect on what these substances added to or detracted from both the New and Old World lifestyles, habits, and diets. The numerous peas, vegetable seeds, and grasses, such as sugarcane, introduced during Columbus' later voyages, made an enormous difference in the lives of New World inhabitants, as did the introduction of the cow and horse, not to mention substances such as coconuts and bananas, that are now intimately associated with the Caribbean and the Bahamas. This article focuses on some of the more important exchange substances and emphasizes many forms of anaphylaxis: asthma, food allergy, hypersensitivity pneumonitis, chronic bronchitis, rhinitis, serum sickness, and other conditions that developed in both New and Old World inhabitants. To mention only a few examples, the Europeans introduced to the New World potential dangers such as honeybees (anaphylaxis). It also gave the New World the cow and the horse (serum sickness), which became the constant companion of Columbus' Indians and the American cowboy. It gave the Italians their thick red gravy, and the New World its pizza (food allergy). The Caribbean received bananas and coconuts and the New World embraced coffee (caffeine addiction). On the other hand, the exchange also caused Europeans to begin puffing away on tobacco!

Columbus' voyages and the exchange of multiple animal products, foods, fowl, grasses, trees, insects, and plants between the New World and the Old, resulted in profound changes in many aspects of life. Among these were changes in dietary habits, manifestation of allergic reactions to new substances, development of habits and addictions to certain substances, introduction of causative agents of new medical ailments, and possible cures for these ailments.

Some of the foods in Columbus' original ship stores are illustrated by a passage from his log on Tuesday, September 4, 1492, as the vessels were being loaded in the Canary Islands: "Today, we loaded and stored dried meat and salted fish and some fruits. The fruit will have to be consumed early, for it will spoil if the voyage is of three weeks' duration. We will load the biscuits tomorrow."[1] Much similar information related to plants, grasses, animals, and fowl, can be gained from reading Columbus' log.[1] Some of this information reveals that as a botanist, ornithologist, and ichthyologist, he was lacking in knowledge. He was however, clearly unsurpassed as a sailor, navigator, and physical scientist

Henderson Professor of Medicine and Vice Chancellor, Tulane University Medical Center, 1430 Tulane Avenue, New Orleans, LA 70112

as evidenced by his mastering of astronomy, meteorology, navigation, and geography.

THE COLUMBIAN EXCHANGE

On Columbus' second voyage in 1493, during which the Europeans became intent on colonizing, he sailed with 17 ships carrying 1200 men, a wide variety of plants, grasses, fruits, and vegetables plus a veritable Noah's Ark of animal species unknown to the newly discovered world. Among these were those animals, grasses, fruits, vegetables, flowering and addictive plants, and medications listed in Table I.

The introduction of these materials seeded large parts of the North American continent with new grasses, such as European bluegrass, and covered large areas of the south with vines, such as kudzu. A variety of Old World diseases introduced by these animals, plants, and the Europeans themselves wreaked havoc on the native population. Europeans also introduced to the New World potential dangers, such as European honeybees, later known as English flies. Indeed, native "Americans" frequently fled whenever they found honeybees in a hollow tree. The bees often advanced ahead of the westward-moving frontier, serving as a reliable sign that Europeans were soon to follow and alerting tribes to move westward ahead of the advancement.[2]

This so-called Columbian Exchange also brought foodstuffs of considerable significance from the newly discovered lands to Europe. Substances that went from the New World to the Old are listed in Table II.

Contrary to popular opinion, the pineapple, which was introduced to Europe at this time, was native to Brazil, Mexico, and the Caribbean islands rather than Hawaii. Other plants like okra were neither European nor native "American" in origin but were later brought to the New World by slaves from Africa, where they had been used in African gumbos. Most of these items came from the southern parts rather than the northern parts of the New World.

The lengthy lists of important substances exchanged between the two worlds is formidable, and it takes little imagination to realize what such foods and substances added to (or perhaps, in the case of tobacco, detracted from) the European lifestyle, habits, and diet.

The New World also benefited greatly from many of the substances introduced from Europe. For example, when introduced to the Caribbean on Columbus' later voyages, the numerous vegetable seeds, wheat, chickpeas, and sugarcane made an enormous difference to the diet and health of later New World inhabitants. Kentucky and Tennessee were seeded with beautiful European bluegrass. The introduction of the cow to the Americas as well as bananas, rice, coffee, coconuts, breadfruit, and a variety of citrus fruits to South America and Brazil was also of considerable dietary and economic significance. Indeed, one can scarcely imagine the Caribbean or the Bahamas without coconuts, bananas, or coffee introduced from Europe.

An entry in Columbus' log, on his discovery of Cuba, notes that the island was very beautiful and filled with flowers, fruits, green trees, and many birds. He described the grass being "as tall as it is in Andalucia in the months of April and May" and claimed to have found a considerable amount of purslane (a herb used to prepare salads), plus a wild amaranth (pigweed).[1] He described cotton growing in the mountains as "the size of large trees" and the land as very different from that of Spain, being covered with panic grass (panizo, a synonym for millet).[1] Many who followed Columbus also noted the aroma of trees and flowers in the New World; some were awed by the smell of giant magnolias. On later voyages, DeSoto's men admired "the very savory, palatable, and fragrant" strawberries in what is now the southeastern part of the United States. Thus, the different varieties of grasses, trees, and their aromas clearly made a distinct impression on the newly arrived Europeans.

We shall focus on a few of the more important exchange substances and attempt to show how they

TABLE I

Old World to the New World

Animals and Fowl	Grasses, Grains, and Nuts	Vegetables	Fruits	Flowers and Plants
Horses	Wheat	Cabbage	Pear	Gladioli
Cows	Rice	Turnips	Peach	Lilac
Sheep	Barley	Lettuce	Lemon	Dandelion
Pigs	Crab grass		Orange	Carnation
Chickens	European blue grass		Banana	Daffodil
Honey bee	Chick peas		Breadfruit	Tulip
	Coconut		Olive	Daisy
				Coffee

TABLE II

New World to the Old World

Grasses and Tubers	Nuts	Flowering Plants and Trees	Fowl	Plants	Peppers	Beans
Corn	Avocado	Sunflower	Turkey	Tobacco	Red	Lima
Potato	Peanut	Petunia		Cacao	Green	Butter
Sweet potato	Pecan	Black-eyed susan		Quinine	Chili	Navy
Pumpkin	Cashew	Marigold		Chewing gum		Kidney
Tomato		Zinnia		Pineapple		
		Poinsettia		Vanilla		
		Dahlia		Cotton		
		Rubber		Cassava		

affected the nutritional and dietary habits and the immune response of the inhabitants of Europe and the New World.

Grasses: Corn.

The impact of the discovery of one variety of grass, namely corn, was of far-reaching importance to the Europeans. Maize, or "mahiz," a variant of its original Taino name, had been cultivated in Mexico for approximately 10,000 years. It was perhaps Columbus' most important plant discovery and the most important of all "new" foodstuffs sent to Europe. Being unfamiliar with the plant, he called it a strange kind of grass. The mahiz in Aztec civilizations were essentially based on maize as a foodstuff. Indeed, maize was the very central crop of the Americas. After its initial introduction into Europe, however, it was grown only as fodder for animals and was not used as a food until much later. In addition to foodstuffs, many valuable products are made from corn (i.e., corn oil and alcoholic beverages). Local Indians in the New England area also introduced it to the pilgrims in seventeenth century North America. They simply referred to it as "corn," a generic word referring to any kind of grain product. Thus, in later years, the pilgrims and subsequent settlers called it "Indian corn."

By the time Columbus first sighted the Bahamas, the inhabitants of many areas of the New World had developed more than 200 varieties of corn, or maize, a remarkable plant-breeding achievement. On his return, Columbus carried some specimens to Europe, and the Spaniards distributed them to many areas surrounding the Mediterranean. The Venetians cultivated many varieties of corn and introduced them to the Near East from where they were sent to the Balkans and often back to the countries of Western Europe.[3]

As a result of Magellan's voyages in the early sixteenth century, corn was known in parts of the South Pacific, particularly the Philippines. The Portuguese introduced corn farming to their African colonies and cultivated it to provide food for the slave trade. It is ironic that a food as cheap as corn constituted an important crop used to feed African slaves on their way to the New World. It is also ironic and tragic that its introduction into Africa and its widespread cultivation resulted in a larger, healthier African population, ensuring more human cargo for slavers.

For the allergist, corn, although not an important allergen, has been documented as a cause of anaphylactic reactions.[4] Some have claimed that corn is a significant food allergen, but this is not the impression of the vast majority of allergists. In one study of 68 children with suspected food allergy in whom double-blind food challenges were performed, none reacted to corn.[5] Mycotoxins, especially aflatoxins and trichothecnes, are important products of many molds and are produced by a wide variety of nuts and corn. Aflatoxins for example, may induce symptoms such as weight loss or loss of appetite but rarely liver disease or carcinoma. Other mycotoxins can induce headache, vertigo, nausea, vomiting, or visual disturbances. Contamination of cereal crops with toxins has resulted in epidemics of postischemic inflammation and even gangrene of limbs. Fortunately, these mycotoxin problems can be prevented by surveillance and destruction of infested crops.[5]

Sugarcane.

This grass probably was cultivated initially in India and Southeast Asia. By the Renaissance period, sugarcane was grown in North Africa, the Canary Islands, and parts of Spain using slave labor. Thus, it was well known to Columbus before his first voyage to the Americas. Sugar, during those times, was essentially a luxury often purchased by Europeans from apothecaries to add to various medicines to improve their taste. After Columbus transported a few pieces of sugarcane to the Caribbean and it became widely cultivated in the New World, the plant flourished rapidly. By the mid-sixteenth century, large forested areas in Brazil and other parts of South America were being destroyed and transformed into ever-increasing colonies of sugarcane plantations. Slave trading and sugarcane growing also became interdependent soon after discovery of the New World. The Spanish, whose original interest was in spices and foods, became preoccupied with gold and silver, leaving the Portuguese to profit, particularly in Brazil, by operating the highly profitable sugarcane plantations with slave labor from Africa. The Portuguese actually acquired papal authority for their undertakings (Nicholas V had given them leave and ordered them to "reduce to perpetual slavery the Saracens, pagans, and other enemies of Christ southward from the Capes Badajor and Non, including all the coast of Guinea").[5] Holland and other countries occupied portions of Northern Brazil to engage in producing the lucrative sugarcane crop. The Dutch then passed along their knowledge of plantation management to the English, French, and Danes, who each acquired several Caribbean islands for sugarcane cultivation. The demand for slaves continued to increase, and labor-intensive cultivation of sugarcane eventually spread to the North American mainland where cotton and tobacco succeeded sugar as plantation-grown crops.

As had been the case in Brazil, large sections of the Caribbean islands were deforested for sugarcane cultivation. The islands became so valuable that the British considered giving up the whole of Canada for the right to hold on to Jamaica; the Dutch agreed to cede New York to England in exchange for the sugar islands of Surinam; France abandoned segments of Canada to the British to hold on to the rich sugarcane plantations of Guadeloupe. A vicious cycle was established whereby slaves were imported to grow sugarcane crops. In turn, some sugar was distilled to produce rum, which was sold in many areas of the world including the New England colonies, and provided increasing revenues to import more African slaves to grow more sugarcane.[4]

This colorful history notwithstanding, the role of sugar is minimal with regard to its possible allergenic properties. Cane sugar has been thought by some to represent one of many causes of headache, although this has not been substantiated. The possible effects on behavior, particularly of children, by abnormal sugar metabolism and high sugar content diets have been the subject of considerable controversy. Some studies have attempted to correlate high sugar intake with lower academic achievement in children. An abnormal glucose tolerance test was reported in some adults with forms of antisocial behavior. Others have attempted to link aggressive and hyperactive behavior in children to sugar rich diets, in the belief such behavior reflects some type of "sugar allergy" or "reactive hypoglycemia." Current research findings refute these mechanistic claims and cast serious doubt on the existence of sugar-induced behavioral disorders.[4]

Bagassosis (a form of hypersensitivity pneumonitis, or allergic alveolitis, involving the lung interstitium, terminal bronchioles, and alveoli first discovered in the New World in 1939)[5] is a potentially disabling pulmonary disease resulting from the inhalation of actinomycete-contaminated sugarcane fiber residue. The acute form of the disease is characterized by recurrent bouts of dyspnea, cough, malaise, chills, and fever several hours after exposure to the fiber residue. A chronic form of the disease with insidious onset of symptoms also exists. The disease has, on occasion, proved to be rampant, occurring in sporadic outbreaks, in certain well-localized areas of the New World.[6] Clinical and animal model studies have demonstrated the importance of T cell and immune complex-mediated pulmonary injury in the disease. This and other forms of hypersensitivity pneumonitis in pigeon breeders, chicken and turkey workers, and in persons inhaling porcine and other animal protein, are all the result of the importation of these substances either into the New World from Europe or vice versa.

Hypersensitivity pneumonitis also results from the inhalation of other organic and vegetable dusts, particularly moldy hay made from many grasses, and can result in the disease called farmers lung.[7] A wide variety of organic dusts from various woods that have been imported from one continent to the other also has caused hypersensitivity pneumonitis in both new and old world inhabitants.

Trees and Plants

Rubber. One tree of note for the allergist is the rubber tree, which was native to the Amazonian rain forests of South America and later imported to Malaya and the Far East. Natural raw latex, the milky sap of the rubber tree, today has multiple uses: in surgical gloves, catheters, condoms, balloons, adhesives, elastic thread, and rubber bands. Many rubber products, including gloves worn by surgeons, dentists, and nurses, pose a very large allergic problem: latex is an example of an "equipment hazard" for medical workers and their patients. Allergy to rubber constituents (polypeptides in natural latex) or rubber additives (phenylenediamine, mercaptobenzothiazole, thiurams, carbamates) can result in contact urticaria, angioedema, inhalant allergies, and unexpected anaphylactic shock. These conditions are being reported with increasing frequency. As of this writing, more than 275 latex-associated anaphylactic reactions with over a dozen deaths have been reported to the Food and Drug Administration. Thus, latex also is an example of a substance originating in the New World that has sensitized large numbers of inhabitants of both the New and Old Worlds.[8]

Cotton. During exploration of Cuba between October 28 and December 5, 1492,[1] Columbus claimed to have seen large numbers of cotton plants growing in mountain areas, often reaching the size of tall trees. This native New World plant was destined to replace sugar as the most lucrative of all crops. The cultivation of cotton actually propagated slavery because, as was sugarcane, it was grown on the plantation system.

The benefits of cotton to mankind in the form of textile manufacturing (clothing, bedding, fabrics, furniture covering, draperies, etc.) have been of inestimable value. It should however, be remembered that a form of occupational lung disease or occupational asthma, namely byssinosis, has caused considerable health problems in cotton workers throughout the world. Byssinosis is a respiratory disease affecting cotton textile mill workers characterized by chest tightness, cough, and dyspnea, usually on the first day of return to work after time off.[9] A more chronic form of cotton dust-induced respiratory disease resembling chronic bronchitis also has been described and is associated with permanent disability. The heterogeneity of cotton dust has not permitted a clear understanding of both the etiologic agent(s) or the pathogenetic mechanisms of byssinosis.[10] Cotton dust itself is defined as dust generated into the atmosphere through processing cotton fibers combined with any naturally occurring materials such as stems, leaves, bracts, and inorganic matter that may have accumulated on the cotton fibers during the growing or harvesting period.[11]

In addition to byssinosis, other health problems likely associated with cotton fiber can affect mill workers. Predominant among these is mill fever, a disease affecting new workers and presenting as chills, fever, and malaise. Tolerance is eventually acquired, and there are no known chronic effects of this illness. The exact prevalence of mill fever in employees is unknown, but estimates range from a low of 10% to a high of 80%.

Tobacco. As early as October 15, 1492, entry in his log (only 3 days after he had landed), Columbus noted of the New World inhabitants that "They brought us parrots, balls of cotton, threads, spears, and many other things, including a kind of dry leaf that they hold in great esteem."[1] Thus, Columbus provided the first account of what would become a global habit. Before this, tobacco had been unknown in Europe, Asia, or Africa. When Columbus reported Caribbean Indians strolling along with "a fire brand in the hand, and herbs to drink the smoke thereof," what he saw were likely cigars. Other Spaniards reported Indians who lit one end of a rolled leaf and inhaled the smoke through a nostril. Mainland Indians puffed pipes, a practice soon copied from England to Japan. Although King James I of England loathed tobacco as a "stinking weed" harmful to the brain and dangerous to the lungs, his addicted subjects made it the number one product of England's American colonies and began cultivating it in Virginia in 1612. Even though unenthused, Thomas Jefferson grew the weed, although he called it "a culture produc-

tive of infinite wretchedness that exhausted the land, as well as the people." Nonetheless, in a little more than 100 years, all of Western Europe was puffing away. Today, tobacco is the most widely distributed of all cultivated plants.

The obvious evils of tobacco for mankind, including its association with chronic bronchitis, asthma, emphysema, carcinoma of the lung, coronary artery disease, Buerger's disease, and other conditions, have been the subject of hundreds of medical and scientific articles and books.[12-14] These health conditions also have been evident in the populations of both the New and Old Worlds for many years.

Beans, Tomatoes, and Peppers

Beans. Before Columbus' voyages, Europe had no bean crops except, possibly, the broad bean. All others, including red and string beans, came from America as did squashes, pumpkins, and gourds. "Pellagra" was rare in South and Central America because the nutrition deficiencies in maize were remedied by adding tomatoes, beans, and fish to the diet. It is of interest that "refrito" beans (a specialty of Mexico today that are boiled, mashed, fried, and topped with grated cheese) evolved only after the Spaniards had introduced the cow and other domesticated animals to Central America. Before that time, there was no reliable supply of fat or oil.

Tomatoes. The tomato was first noted as a weed in prehistoric times, but by the time Cortez and his 400 Spaniards reached Mexico in 1519, it had been carefully cultivated and had increased enormously in yield and variety. Cortez was impressed with the many varieties of tomato under cultivation by the Aztecs and their incorporation in many dishes. The first tomatoes introduced into Europe in the sixteenth century were probably of an orange-yellow variety, which would account for one of their Early European names, "golden apple." The Spaniards called them "tomate" (from the Aztec word "tomatl") and adopted them readily into their diet. Italy also acquired a taste for tomatoes sometime later[15] when a Jesuit priest brought a red variety to Europe from America. A few decades later, tomato sauce, an enormously successful complement to pasta, made its first appearance. One cannot imagine today's Italian cuisine without it. Yet, despite its success in Italy and Europe in general, tomatoes were rejected as a food source by early North American settlers until the mid-nineteenth century because they were thought to be poisonous and merely ornamental.

Peppers. There has always been confusion over the classification and names of peppers. In general, the multisized chili peppers are used to season foods. Their flavor is "very hot," and the seeds can actually burn mucosal tissues. Some are dried and ground to make powders, such as cayenne pepper, and others are pickled in vinegar to make Tabasco and other types of Louisiana hot sauces. The familiar large green, yellow, and red bell peppers are used in salads or vegetable dishes. Other varieties are used to make paprika, a mild spice without the sharp, hot pungency of chili peppers.

It should be remembered that one of Columbus' prime objectives was to discover new peppers and spices on his voyages. One such spice discovered by Columbus was the Central American capsicum pepper that bore no relationship to the piper nigrum of India. Capsicum is the pungent compound in hot red peppers that is best known for its ability to stimulate neuropeptide release from nonmyelevated afferent vagal fibers. This can result in sneezing, locomotion, cough, changes in airway caliber (wheezing), vascular tone mucus release, and vascular permeability.

The Spaniards were quick to apply the old name "pimienta" to the hot-tasting capsicums found in Mexico. The people of tropical America still use capsicums (dried, pickled, powdered, etc.) when preparing nearly all foods. In early post-Columbian times, capsicums went into soups, stews, sauces, and vegetable preparations. In early seventeenth century Mexico, it was estimated that there were at least 40 varieties of capsicums; currently there are 92.[16]

Vanilla. Vanilla is actually a member of the orchid family that produces a greenish-yellow flower. Native to Southern Mexico and Central America, the pod is used as a spice. The Aztecs used vanilla to concoct drinks that were offered to Cortez by their chieftains.

Roots: Potatoes and Other Tubers

Potato. When Francisco Pizarro went south from the Caribbean into Peru, he was confronted by a people who had a richness of food with an abundance of fish, deer, wild llama, bear, puma, fox, and a large rodent called "vizecacha." Ducks were domesticated and guinea pigs were raised in households. Most Peruvian food was vegetarian: squash, beans, sweet potatoes, peanuts, tomatoes, potatoes, chili peppers, and maize. Potatoes, unlike the peanut, were entirely new to the Spaniards, who originally encountered them in Haiti and later introduced them into Malaysia and China. At elevations above 11,000 feet in Peru, where maize does not grow well, the main crops consisted of potatoes and other related tubers. The potato had become a popular food for the Peruvians, and they developed a method of freezing and repeatedly drying them to store for long periods.

The Spaniards considered potatoes "a dainty dish"[17] and brought the vegetable to Europe in 1570 where it was rapidly cultivated and became a basic food for their ship stores. Initially, however, Europeans, who essentially ate grains rather than root crops, considered the potato, like the tomato, to be an ornamental plant because of its purple flowers. All sorts of attributes were

assigned to the potato in Europe where it was described as "very substantial, good and restorative." It also was claimed that eating potatoes could stop "fluxes of the bowels," cure consumption, and "increase seed and provoke lust, causing fruitfulness in both sexes."[17] In Burgundy, however, potatoes were banned in 1619 because they were believed to cause leprosy when frequently eaten. According to Diderot's *Encyclopédie,* "However it is prepared, this root [the potato] is tasteless and starchy." As late as the mid-1700s, the French primarily used potatoes as fodder for animals and food only for peasants.[4] Benjamin Rumford, in designing a diet to feed the poor as well and as cheaply as possible, concluded that barley soup thickened with potatoes and peas, seasoned with vinegar, and served with pieces of stale bread to promote chewing, was ideal for this purpose.[18] The poor were, however, quite resistant to eating potatoes, and it was some time before they could be persuaded to even taste Rumford's soup. In Russia, for example, the government's 1940 order to peasants to plant potatoes met with great resistance, resulting in riots in ten provinces.[19]

Except in countries such as Ireland, where the potato became popular soon after its introduction, it took essentially 200 years for the potato to become widely distributed. The potato was eventually returned to Virginia by English settlers on the eastern US coast and later by the Irish during their mass immigration during Ireland's potato famine.

Potato crops first failed in Ireland in 1845 with potatoes rotting in the fields. The crop failure spread from Ireland to Scotland and on to France, Germany, and Poland, seriously affecting the diets of peasants in countries dependent on the potato as a food source. In Ireland, and to a lesser extent in Scotland, the result was famine, a disaster equal in magnitude to the great plagues.[4] Ordinarily, potato crops and the land on which they grew were not ruined (as was grain) during land battles or raids by pirates and soldiers because they remained hidden below the surface during the winter. A tiny cottage plot could produce enough to feed a man, his wife, their many children, plus their animals. During one catastrophic month in 1845, however, crops throughout Europe began to wilt and rot as potato blight pathogens and spores devoured the sap and killed the plants. This resulted not only in the scarcity of the potato as a food source but in an absence of seed potatoes from which to grow the next year's crop. The net result was severe hunger followed by scurvy, brought on by the lack of vitamin C that potatoes supplied. Later symptoms involved the nervous system and eyes, resulting from a shortage of vitamins A and B. Cow's milk would have provided the necessary vitamins, but when the food source disappeared, the cows died off. One and one-half million Irishmen died, and an equivalent number left Ireland forever and immigrated to the United States and Europe. New disease-resistant strains grown in the New World were later reintroduced into Europe, and the crop was reestablished, emphasizing the importance of preserving wild plant species.

Sweet Potatoes. Columbus described Cuba as having very fertile, well-cultivated land with abundant niames (the common sweet potato), beans "very different from ours", and panic grass (panizo, a synonym for millet). In a log entry dated Sunday, December 16, 1492, he notes that the country is very cool and high and postulates that "Upon the highest mountain plowing could be done with oxen and everything could be transformed into fields and pastures." The fields were planted mostly with ajes (a word used by the Tiano to describe tubers that Columbus says are identical to the niames). Columbus wrote that the ajes somewhat resembled carrots or "cooked roots that had the flavor of chestnuts"[20] and that the Indians served them as bread by grating and kneading the tubers and baking them in a fire.[1] Bread made from the ajes is called "cacabi." Columbus also notes that there are two or three kinds of ajes. These are the first historical notes of plants previously unknown to Europeans, namely manihot esculenta, and ipomoea batatas. To these species and their varieties he applied the only word he knew for a large edible root, namely niame. By the mid-sixteenth century, the English corruption of the term "niame" or "name" changed it to "yam" (the true yam is a native of Africa and belongs to a different family of plants).

Today, we know each of the roots and tubers that Columbus described by different names. manihot esculenta is known in English as yuca or cassava and tapioca. Manioc is Brazilian in derivation. Yuca is a Taino word for one of the varieties, and cassava (cazabe in Spanish) is the Taino word for bread (cacabi) made from the plant. Tapioca is a Brazilian name for the food of the same name made from the plant. It is also widely used as a general name in India.

In the December 16 log entry,[1] Columbus described the ipomoea batatas, one of the more than 400 species in the morning glory family, known to us as the sweet potato. Batata was the name used for the sweet potato, in the region of Santo Domingo. Later, the Spaniards applied a corruption of batata (patata) to the white potato (found in the Andes). Eventually, the English corrupted this to potato. To further confuse things, the English then borrowed the Afro-Hispanic word "niame," changed it to "yam," and applied it to the sweet potato. On his return to Europe, Columbus' ships were laden with sweet potatoes and cassava, which his crew members detested.

Chocolate and Coffee

Chocolate. Another of the New World's important gifts to the Old was chocolate. Cacau, or cocoa, although primarily an African crop at present, was native to southern Mexico and Central America. The natives whipped a concoction of chocolate, maize, and chili peppers into a frothy drink.

Although many New World foods could be grown in Europe, the tropical cacau tree could not, except for the warmer Spanish and Portuguese territories. Hence, the production and consumption of cocoa remained a guarded monopoly for many years.

Chocolate drinks were made by drying cocoa beans, roasting them, and pounding them with water. Occasionally powdered flowers or sugar were added. In Mexico, this chocolate paste was mixed with spices and shaken in a gourd until it frothed. It was then gulped down in one swallow "with admirable pleasure and satisfaction of the bodily nature to which it gives strength, nourishment, and vigor."[21]

The preparation of a pot of chocolate was a complex operation in Spain consisting of mixing the chocolate with chili or peppercorns and certain flowers. Instead of the flowers, one could also use rose powder, logwood dye, cinnamon, various nuts, sugar, and a yellowish orange dye known as annatto.[22]

By the early 1600s, chocolate was exported to Italy, France, and England, and a chocolate house was opened in London in 1657, with the approval of Pepys. Chocolate remained exclusively a drink for several hundred years after its introduction into Europe, and it was not until 1870 that the Swiss invented milk chocolate in solid block form for eating.

Coffee. Contrary to popular belief, coffee actually originated in Ethiopia, a part of the Old World. All New World coffee trees are actually descendants of a single tree cultivated in the botanical garden of seventeenth century Amsterdam. There are many myths about who discovered that it was drinkable. The word itself derives from the Turkish "kahveh" and the Arabic "qahwah," which originally meant wine. Coffee is, indeed, a wine of the Muslims, to whom real wine is forbidden.[4] The people of Constantinople, for example, honored guests with "a cup of coffee, made of a kind of seed called coava, and of a blackish color; which they drink as hot as they possibly can."[23] Encountering it in Persia in the 1620s, Sir Thomas Herbert described coffee as "a drink imitating that in the Stygian Lake, black, thick and bitter."[24]

When it arrived in England in 1657, coffee was hailed as a wholesome drink that "closes the oriface of the stomack, fortifies the heat within, helpeth digestion, quickeneth the spirits, maketh the heart lightsom, is good against eye-sores, coughs or colds, rhumes, consumption, head-ach, dropsie, gout, scurrvey, kings evil and many others" (London Publick Advisor, May 19, 1657).[4] Its introduction into the New World (Brazil, Columbia, Costa Rica), Southeast Asia, and the West Indies vastly increased the world's crop. Coffee cultivation in these countries illustrates that when a nation's economy is based on a simple, profitable export crop, social conditions, political climates, and local labor markets are profoundly affected.

Insects, Lizards, and Worms

Exotic foods. Some foods eaten by the natives gave the conquistadors cause for concern because of their exotic nature, especially those drawn from around or in the many lakes in the new Americas. Tropical America has always been short of animal food, so there existed a tradition of eating local insects found in or near streams and ponds. In addition to conventional pond life, such as frogs and small fish, water flies, large fat spiders, tadpoles, larva, white worms that breed in rotten wood, winged ants, crabs and a large tree lizard (the iguana), which even Columbus' sailors thought to be "white, soft, and tasty,"[20] all served as exotic native foodstuffs. Another luxury, the agave worm, or maguey slug (meocuilin), was often served with guacamole, which even in Aztec times was made with tomatoes, capsicums, and avocados. This worm was a great delicacy at the Aztec court and remains so today in Mexico.

Human Flesh. The Carib Indians were known to be cannibalistic toward their Arawak neighbors, and Columbus claimed to have taken several Caribs to Spain to prevent them from eating their neighbors. The Caribs believed that men could increase their strength by literally consuming the strength of a worthy adversary in battle. Ceremonial cannibalism came as a profound culture shock to the Spaniards. It was said that the Carib Indians were connoisseurs of human flesh and prepared it by cutting the body into various pieces, much like a European butcher.[25] According to one apocryphal story by a Frenchman: The French were delicious, the English so-so, the Dutch tasteless, and the Spanish tough and virtually inedible. It was the tough Spaniards, whose translation of the word Carib into Calib and then Canib, who gave us the derivation of the word cannibal.

According to Aztec rationale of the rite of blood sacrifice, their gods insisted on being appeased by having the living heart of the sacrificial victim presented before them. Aztec priests would often use prisoners of war, literally ripping them open alive and pulling the still-beating hearts from their chests. After the head was hung on a skull rack, part of the body was burned in a fire that was presented to the supreme council of priests. The remainder of the body was returned to the victim's captor, who cooked it at home into something called "tlacatlaolli" (maize and man stew) that was eaten by the entire family. Young puppies were also considered to be a gourmet's delicacy for certain of the Indian tribes, whereas other tribes abhorred eating dog meat.

Barbecue and Baked Seafood. Early American settlers also learned from the Indians how to have a seacoast clam bake: dig a pit, line it with flat stones and light a fire on them, brush away the embers and replace them with layers of seaweed interspersed with layers of clams and ears of maize. From Caribbean sources the colonists acquired methods of barbecuing and smoking dry meat on wood lattices constructed over fires of animal bones and hides. The Caribs called this technique "boucan," which was adopted into the French language as "boucanier" or "buccaneers," a term used to describe outcast shipwrecked sailors and other runaways often took refuge on the Caribbean Islands and "barbecued" captured animals as a means of sustenance.

NATIVE AMERICAN DOMESTIC LIVESTOCK

Mexico's only domesticated livestock were the turkey and the dog, the latter being regarded as a useful, but inferior, meat. After the arrival of the conquistadors and the introduction of the cow from Europe, the dog lost some of its usefulness as a food animal. The turkey became more popular and reached England soon after its first arrival in Europe in the early sixteenth century through the Levantines (Turkish merchants who usually stopped off at Seville on trips to and from the Eastern Mediterranean). Because they were not familiar with the Mexican name for the bird (Uexolotol), they probably could not pronounce it well. The English simply called the bird "turkie cock."[26] There was some confusion between turkey and guinea fowl, which was brought to Europe from West Africa by the Portuguese, but this problem was soon clarified. It is noteworthy that no other nations of the Old World called the bird a "turkey" except the Egyptians. There was general confusion over its name in other areas of Europe where it was attributed to India in keeping with the term applied to the New World (the New Indies) long after the error had been discovered. Despite the confusion, one thing is certain: the turkey established itself quickly and firmly on most Old World dining tables.

OTHER NEW WORLD FISH, BIRDS, AND BEASTS

Columbus reported that

Other than parrots, I have seen no beast of any kind. . . . Here the fishes are so unlike ours, that it is amazing. There are some like dorados, of the brightest colors in the world—blue, yellow, red, multi-colored in a thousand ways; and the colors are so bright that anyone would marvel and take a great delight at seeing them. Also, there are whales. I have seen no land animals of any sort, except parrots and lizards—although a boy told me that he saw a big snake. I have not seen sheep, goats, or any other beasts. . . While going around one of the lagoons I saw a serpent, which we killed with lances, and I am bringing Your Highnesses the skin. When it saw us, it went into the lagoon, and we followed it in because the water is not very deep. This serpent is about 6 feet long. I think there are many rich serpents in these lagoons. The people here eat them and the meat is white and taste like chicken.[1]

The serpent to which he referred was an iguana.

In his November 6, 1492, entry, Columbus describes the many birds on the island as being totally different from those of Spain, except for the partridge and the nightingale. He also describes seeing a great number of geese, but again, no four-footed beasts, other than "dogs that do not bark" (perhaps a reference to raccoons).

OLD WORLD HORSES AND PIGS

In 1493, when the 17 ships of the expedition landed and unloaded Columbus' 2 dozen mares and stallions, the Indians were amazed at the strange creatures and thought that they were the biggest dogs they had ever seen. Surely, they reasoned, they must be dogs, since only dogs walked on four legs and got along with people. It is known that horses had inhabited the Americas during the Pleistocene era but vanished along with the saber-toothed tigers and mastodons only to return 10,000 years later with Columbus and Spanish conquistadors. Columbus' horses were referred to as "sky dogs" by the Aztecs, who thought that each rider and horse represented one huge godlike creature. These sky dogs propagated rapidly and, within a century, herds ran wild from North America to Argentina. Needless to say, the horses made it easier for Indian tribes to hunt buffalo and other game. The diets and lifestyles of the native Americans also improved as did their ability to use the horse to resist the relentless advancement of Europeans.[27]

Columbus never kept track of the eight pigs that he took to the Caribbean settlement of Hispaniola in 1493, but one Diego Vaslasquez De Cullar saw what happened to the 2 dozen he unloaded in Cuba in 1498. Within 16 years, the pigs increased to 30,000. Hogs were seeded on nearly every island, reproducing at an average rate of three big litters a year, guaranteeing a steady supply of protein for Old World immigrants. The pigs also altered the fundamental ecology of the Caribbean by their eating habits.[27]

MEDICATIONS

In addition to food allergies, anaphylactic reactions from foreign proteins, asthma, rhinitis, hypersensitivity pneumonitis, and exchanges of various herbs and "medications" markedly affected the population. For example, the willow bark was among the herbal remedies of the New World. This bark is, of course, known to contain salicin, the drug used in the synthetic form in aspirin.

The medicine quinine, derived from the bark of the cinchona tree that dotted the slopes of the Peruvian Andes, is important in that it enabled Old World Europeans to colonize the tropics and develop empires in Asia and Africa in the nineteenth century. This Indian cure for malaria even helped Abraham Lincoln win the Civil War. Union troops had plentiful supplies of quinine, but the Confederacy had been deprived of this wonder drug by Union blockade, resulting in the loss of many men to malarial fevers. The effect of herbs, medications, foods, and other substances imported from the New World was felt not only in Europe but also in Africa. For example, quinine was used in Africa to treat malaria.

CONCLUSIONS

It is obvious that the Columbian Exchange of multiple grasses, trees, plants, pollens, exotic foods, domestic livestocks, fish, birds and other species has had enormous effects on the New and Old Worlds, both beneficial and harmful. Of particular importance to the allergist and clinical immunologist has been the little known and interesting facet of this massive exchange on the host response to a wide variety of these newly introduced foreign substances, namely allergic reactions by inhabitants of both worlds on coming in contact with various new foods, animals, and insect products. These reactions range from simple allergic rhinitis, urticaria, and bronchial asthma on one hand to more severe forms of hypersensitivity pneumonitis and anaphylactic shock on the other.

For example, it can easily be seen that the native American population was subject to anaphylactic reactions from the newly imported European honeybee. Protein from European chickens was not only a source of asthma and rhinitis but hypersensitivity pneumonitis as well. Horse protein was a potent allergen in production of rhinitis and asthma. In addition, horses subsequently were used for many years to develop antiserum against tetanus and other organisms. These antisera proved to be another cause of severe anaphylaxis. Cow's milk was an important source of allergens, causing respiratory, gastrointestinal, and pulmonary reactions, particularly in infants and children. Wheat flour was a prelude to baker's asthma and certain forms of occupational allergy, which are of considerable importance in today's industrialized society.

The European bluegrass that seeded much of the central plain areas was a potent source of allergen for spring and summer rhinitis and asthma. Clearly, proteins in nuts (peanuts, pecans, cashews, Brazilian nuts, and sunflower seeds) are important causes of life-threatening anaphylaxis, angioedema, and urticaria. They must have added to the burden of allergens causing such systemic reactions in the European population.

Likewise, proteins and other constituents of turkeys can cause rhinitis and asthma and are reported to cause hypersensitivity pneumonitis in those who raise birds for commercial purposes. The introduction of tobacco into Europe had enormous effects on its population. Tobacco leaf is known to cause occupational asthma in leaf workers, and its incineration products are well-known to be important risk factors in the production of emphysema, chronic bronchitis, and bronchogenic carcinoma; it is also a respiratory tract irritant. Animal proteins from the pig cause anaphylactic reactions and upper respiratory symptoms. Porcine pituitary extract, when insufflated as a form of treatment for diabetes insipidus, is known to cause hypersensitivity pneumonitis. In addition to other foods known to cause anaphylactic reactions, virtually all the common vegetables imported into Europe from the New World (i.e., corn, tomatoes, various types of beans, and others) are known to cause food allergies manifested by diarrhea, urticaria, angioedema, gastrointestinal cramps, or related symptoms, thus adding to the overall burden of allergens thrust upon the European population as a result of Columbus' voyages. The same can be said for other vegetable and citrus products such as lemons, oranges, peaches, pears, rice, barley, and others imported from the Old World to the New World.

Corn, an American staple for thousands of years, markedly enhanced African diets, boosting the continent's birthrates and life spans. The same can be said for the potato, which fed and improved the livelihood of millions of peasants in European countries, particularly Ireland, Scotland, Germany, Poland, and which was ultimately transported back to the New World after disease ruined European potato crops in the 1840s.

Whether Columbus is seen as a great discoverer or as merely a rapacious messenger of all good tidings who wreaked havoc on a peaceful, relatively advanced agrarian society, it must be admitted that the exchange of these substances between the two worlds and the result of these effects constituted one of the most important events in human history.

REFERENCES

1. Fuson RH. The Log of Christopher Columbus. Camden, ME: International Marine Publishing Co., 1987.
2. America before Columbus; the Columbian Exchange, U.S. News World Report. July 9, 1991, p. 26.
3. Settipane GA. Latex allergy: Another occupational risk for physicians. Allergy Proc 13:79, 1992.
4. Tannahill R. Food in History. New York: Crown Publishers, Inc., 1989.
5. National Institutes of Health Publication 84-2442. Adverse Reactions to Foods. July 1984, p. 44.
6. Salvaggio JE, Buechner HA, Seabury JH, Arquembourg PC. Bagassosis I: Precipitins against extracts of crude bagasse in the serum of patients. Ann Intern Med 64:748–758, 1966.
7. Salvaggio JE, Arquembourg PC, Seabury JH, Buechner HA. Bagassosis IV: Precipitins against extracts of thermophilic actinomycetes in patients with bagassosis. Am J Med 46:538–544, 1969.
8. Salvaggio JE. Hypersensitivity pneumonitis. In: Slavin R, Ed. Tice Practice of Medicine, I. Philadelphia, PA: Harper & Row, 1971.
9. O'Neil CE, Butcher BT, Reed MA, Salvaggio JE. In vitro effects of aqueous cotton dust extract on leukocyte cyclic adenosine monophosphate levels. Agents Actions 14:210–215, 1984.
10. O'Neil CE, Butcher BT, Salvaggio JE. Mechanisms in byssinosis: A review. In: Montalvo JG, Ed. ACS Symposium on Cotton Dust, 1982, pp. 145–162.
11. Butcher BT, O'Neil CE, Jones RN. The respiratory effect of cotton dust. Clin Chest Med 4:63–70, 1983.
12. Harris CC. Tobacco smoke and lung disease: Who is susceptible? Ann Intern Med 105:607–608, 1986.
13. Smoking and Health: A report of the Surgeon General. Part I-II. Involuntary Smoking. Washington, DC: Government Printing Office, 1979. (DHEW publication PHS 79-50066).
14. Repace JL, Lowery AH. Indoor air pollution, tobacco smoke, and public health. Science 208:464–472, 1980.
15. Coats AM. The fruit with a shady past. County Life May 1973, p. 17.
16. Ucko PJ, Dimbleby GW, Eds. The Domestication and Exploitation of Plants and Animals. 1969, p. 447.
17. Castellanas Juan de, quoted in Salamon RN, The History and Social Influence of the Potato. 1949, p. 102.
18. Rumford BT. Of food: And particularly of feeding the poor (1795). Works, vol. V. London: Gower Publishers 1876, p. 403.
19. Smith REF, Christian D. Bread and Salt: A Social and Economic History of Food and Drink in Russia. 1984, pp. 280–283.
20. The Life of the Admiral Christopher Columbus; by his son Ferdinand, Keen B, trans. New Brunswick, NJ: Rutgers University Press, 1959.
21. Carletti, Francesco. Ragionementi (1594–1606). trans. Weinstock H, My Voyage Around the World; 1964, p. 53.
22. Franklin A. Vie privee des francais, 12e a' 18e siecles. 27 t, Paris 1887–1902. Vo. XIII Le Cafe, le the, et le chocolat. pp. 161–167.
23. Lithgow W. The Total Discourse of the Rare Adventures and Painful Perigrinations of Long Nineteene Yeares Travayles from Scotland to the Most Famous Kingdomes in Europe, Asia and Affrica [1632]. Edinburg: Edinburg Press, 1906, pp. 58–59.
24. Herbert T. Some Yeares Travels into Africa and Asia the Great. 1638. In: Tannahill R. Food in History. New York: Crown Publishers, Inc., 1989, p. 275.
25. Tannahill R. Flesh and Blood: A History of the Cannibal Complex. New York: Crown Publishers, Inc. 1975, p. 76.
26. Powell G. Jahavger's turkey-cock. History Today. December 1970, pp. 857–858.
27. America Before Columbus; the Columbian Exchange, "The Animal that Changed History." U.S. News World Report. July 8, 1991, p. 29. □

Chapter 9

New World Plants; New World Drugs

ABSTRACT

The "discovery" and eventual colonization and exploitation of the New World by Europeans created the opportunity for the development of medicines from numerous plants native to the Western Hemisphere. Many of these plants had been employed by native cultures for centuries or millenia. The plants and, eventually, isolated drugs derived from them were incorporated into the materia medica of the Europeans both in Europe and in the new colonies. Many became official in the United States Pharmacopeia (USP); a few still remain today. In all, 30 plants and/or their derivatives are briefly profiled. The subject of plant-based medicines is becoming more timely as millions of Europeans and Americans begin to seek "natural" remedies for self-medication. Unfortunately, lack of patentability and high new-drug approval costs keep many traditional plant medicines from obtaining proper recognition.

"There are trees of a thousand types, all with their various fruits and all scented. I am the saddest man in the world because I do not recognize them, for I am sure they are of great value in Spain for dyes and as medicinal spices. I am bringing specimens of them to Your Highnesses." Christopher Columbus' journal entries, October 19 and 21, 1492 (Griffenhagen, 1992)

"There are 121 prescription drugs in use today in many different countries in the world that come from only 90 species of plants. Of those, 74 percent came from following up native folklore claims. There are 250,000 species of plants on the planet. A logical person would have to say there are a lot more jackpots out there." Norman R. Farnsworth, Ph.D., Research Professor of Pharmacognosy and Senior University Scholar, University of Illinois at Chicago (Blumenthal, 1992)

"The pharmaceutical industry in the United States has attained in the prescription market alone annual sales in excess of $3 billion from the medicinal agents first discovered in plants, many of them found in use amongst unlettered peoples in aboriginal societies the world around. Can we afford any longer to neglect this prolific and promising treasure-trove of ethnopharmacological knowledge that may not long be available?" Richard Evans Schultes, Ph.D., D.Sc., F.M.L.S, Edward C. Jeffrey Professor of Biology, Emeritus, at Harvard University, former director of the Harvard Botanical Museum (Schultes, 1991)

"Despite decades of enthusiasm in developed countries for chemically synthesized drugs, plants are still a highly important source. Some seven thousand compounds currently used in modern medicine are derived from natural products; most have been used for centuries by European, Asian and Amerindian healers. In 1985 the world market of drugs was estimated at $150 billion; plants accounted for $43 billion of that and represent about a quarter of the active ingredients in prescription drugs." (Elisabetsky, 1990)

It is almost a cliché that Columbus' motivation for initiating his voyages that led to the discovery of the "New World" was prompted by his search for a new water route to the Indies. The economic incentive for such an undertaking was to provide a shorter route to the rich spice-producing islands and coast of India, and to break the stranglehold of Arab merchants whose monopoly on this trade resulted in high prices paid by Europeans for these plant materials. In more contemporary terms, it is as if Columbus was looking for a way to stop the European balance of trade deficit.

Columbus never realized that he had discovered a New World as a result of his three voyages, and he died still believing he had found a new route to the Indies. In fact, on his first voyage, he believed that the indigenous plant he found on what is now known as Cuba, was the mastic tree (*Pistacia lenticus*), the source of the

---

Executive Director, American Botanical Council, Austin, Texas. Editor, HerbalGram

---

Old World drug gum mastic, at that time used as a treatment for diarrhea and cholera. As a possible consequence of Columbus' confusion, the plant he thought was mastic and exported back to Spain under this name, the gumbo-limbo tree (*Bursera simaruba*) is still sometimes called "mastic tree" (Griffenhagen, 1992).

That Columbus' voyages opened up a new source of plants for food and pharmaceutical use is well established. Numerous articles and books have hailed the debt that people the world over owe to New World food crops. Items mentioned among many others, are corn, potatoes (herein spelled properly), tomatoes, pumpkin, squash, wild rice, chocolate, vanilla, capsicum "peppers," pineapple, papaya, and many others (Viola and Margolis, 1991).

New world plants also added to the expanded materia medica of Europe, although some scholars insist that their introduction was constrained by considerable cultural barriers. "The rationale for the therapeutic use of such plants and actual indications vary greatly since each healing system has its own explanatory models developed within specific sociocultural context" (Risse, 1984). Despite such understandable cultural barriers, a number of New World plants gained popularity in Europe. Among those almost always cited as examples of New World drugs are quinine and ipecac. Other accounts include the sarsaparilla root (*Smilax officinalis*), first introduced into Europe as a remedy for syphilis and rheumatism (Lloyd, 1929; Hobbs, 1988).

OFFICIAL DRUGS DERIVED FROM NEW WORLD PLANTS

What follows is a listing of pharmaceutical drugs that have been and/or still are recognized as official medicines in the United States. Some have been discontinued because of safety and efficacy considerations or because more effective pharmaceuticals have replaced them; some still are in use or are of recent introduction. Although this list is not intended to be exhaustive, its aim is to be comprehensive. In each listing the author has attempted to include the drug's generic name, plant source including both Latin name and plant family, common name, original geographic source, and former or current uses.

Finally, this article notes whether the drug has been listed in the United States Pharmacopoeia (USP). Many were subsequently dropped in their crude or extract form in favor of listings for single constituents. After losing official USP status, many drugs were still listed in the National Formulary (NF), but this designation is noted only occasionally herein. The drugs and materia medica are listed alphabetically with the plants Latin binomial in italics and the plant family in parentheses.

Balsam of Peru

Myroxylon balsamum var. *pereirae* (Leguminosae or pea family) The leaves and fruits of this tree have been used in its native Mexico and Central America, and the bitter, acrid, vanilla-smelling resin was employed by natives for asthma, catarrh, rheumatism, and for external wounds. Although not native to the area, "Peruvian balsam" as it has been called, derived its name from its original point of export to Europe from Lima, Peru (Lloyd). It was first employed in Europe in seventeenth century Germany pharmacy (Lloyd). Morton (1977) notes its use as a bactericide, fungicide, and parasiticide in cases of "scabies, ringworm, pediculosis, granulations, superficial ulcerations, wounds, bed sores, diaper rash, and chilblains." It also has been used as an ingredient in dental cements and suppositories. It was formerly used for bronchitis, laryngitis, dysmenorrhea, diarrhea, dysentery, and leucorrhea (Morton, 1977). It has been listed in the USP from 1820 to 1990, although it is no longer used internally. Balsam Peru has been used as a food flavoring and fragrance material.

Balsam of Tolu

Myroxylon balsamum (Leguminosae) This drug is derived from a tree native to Argentina, Paraguay, Brazil, Venezuela, Bolivia, Peru, and Colombia. The name Balsam of Tolu derived from a small town near Cartagena, Colombia, from where the greatest quantities were exported. The balsum formerly was used as antitussive and respiratory, used in lozenges for coughs and sore throat, in cough syrups and pill coatings, and as a heated vapor inhalant for respiratory ailments. It also was an ingredient in tincture of benzoin (Morton, 1977). It was official in the USP from 1820 to 1955. Balsam Tolu has been approved as a safe food flavoring ingredient and is used as fragrance material in perfumery.

Bromelain

Aranas comosus; A sativus (Bromeliaceae) This is an enzyme from pineapple originally found in Brazil and the West Indies. Traditional folk medicine uses include diuretic and, in large quantity, as a promoter of uterine contractions. Bromelain is used as a digestive aid, sometimes combined with pancreatin. It also has been used as an anti-inflammatory agent after dental, gynecological, and general surgery, as well as used in treatment of "sprains, contusions, hematomas, abscesses and ulcerations" (Morton, 1977). Morton also cites a review of bromelain with 304 bibliographic references wherein its uses in dematology, stomatology, urology, gynecology, geriatry, and the treatments of phlebitis and pulmonary edema are discussed.

Capsaicin

Capsicum frutescens, C annuum, etc. (Solanaceae or nightshade family). When the Spanish landed in the New World, they mistakenly thought that capsicum fruits were a form of the "peppercorns" with which they were familiar, the fruits of black pepper (*Piper nigrum*) of the Malabar coast of India. Hence, the misnomer red or cayenne "pepper" still applied to fruits of various capsicum species. Capsaicin is the sesquiterpenoid found in the placenta of the fruits and currently is used in topical skin creams for treatment of herpes lesions and psoriasis. Capsicum was official in the USP from 1820 to 1930.

Cascarosides

Rhamnus purshiana (Rhamnaceae) Cascarasides are anthraquinones derived from the bark of a tree found in northern California and the Pacific Northwest. Cascara bark literally means "sacred bark" as the Spanish noted early native uses. Cascarasides are approved as an active ingredient in over-the-counter (OTC) stimulant laxatives. According to Lloyd, cascara is laxative in small doses; cathartic in large doses. Morton (1977) notes that use of fresh bark can cause griping and nausea. Hence the bark is stored for 6 months to 1 year whereupon chemical changes take place that eliminate these adverse effects. Cascara has been official in the USP from 1890 until present.

Cissampeline

Cissampelos pareira (Menispermaceae, moonseed family) This drug is a bisbenzylisoquinoline alkaloid derived from the vine sometimes referred to as false pareira. From Ecuador and related areas in the American tropics, this drug is a skeletal muscle relaxant and, according to Schultes and Raffauf (1991), is one of the primary components of curare. The plant was traditionally used for diuretic, expectorant, emmenagogue, febrifuge. The roots were reportedly used to prevent threatened abortion, relieve menorrhagia, arrest uterine hemorrhage (Uphof, 1968). Morton (1977) says this plant contains alkaloids with neuromuscular blocking action and has been exported in substitution for roots of *Chondrodendron tomentosum*, source of *d*-turbocurarine (see below).

Cocaine

Erythroxylum coca (Erythroxylaceae) No treatment of plant drugs of the New World would be complete without mention of cocaine, a tropane alkaloid derived from the leaves of the Andean shrub coca. Coca leaves have a long history of use in Bolivia and Peru when chewed by natives for energy, stamina, and ability to work for long periods without hunger. The leaves were first introduced to Europe by the Spanish physician Mondardes in 1569. The alkaloid cocaine, first isolated in 1860 and its value as a local anesthetic was discovered by Koller in 1884 (Der Marderosian and Yelvigi, 1976). It was used traditionally as a stimulant, and appetite suppressant (Morton, 1977). The leaves were official in the USP from 1882 to 1916; the derivative alkaloid cocaine was official in USP from 1905 to 1955, and in the NF from 1955 to the present (Der Marderosian and Yelvigi, 1976).

Copaiba

Copaifera officinalis and related species (Leguminosae or pea family) This drug is a balsam from a tree principally found in Venezuela and Brazil. Copaiba was used as a urinary tract disinfectant and has diuretic, stimulant, expectorant, and laxative properties. (Tyler et al., 1988) It was official in the USP from 1820 to the 1910 edition.

Diosgenin

Dioscorea villosa, D composita, D floribunda (Dioscoreaceae) The wild yam, a native of Mexico, constitutes one of the most important sources of plant-derived drugs in the twentieth century. The tuber of the Mexican wild yam was formerly the source for the antifertility steroids first used in birth control pills.. "The steroidal drugs derived from diosgenin include oral contraceptives, anti-inflammatory compounds (topical hormones, systemic corticosteroids), androgens, estrogens, progestogens, and other sex hormone combinations" (Morton, 1977).

Elm Bark

Ulmus fulva; Urubra (Ulmaceae) Elm bark is derived from the inner bark of the slippery elm tree native to the eastern and central United States from Canada to the south. The mucilaginous inner bark formerly was used by natives as a poultice for wounds (Lloyd, 1929) and has been used in medicine for its demulcent, emollient, and antitussive properties (*British Herbal Pharmacopoeia*) for use in stomach ulcers and in cough lozenges (Morton, 1977). The bark was official in the USP from 1820 through the 1910 edition and is still approved as an over-the-counter drug ingredient as a demulcent.

Emetine

(See Ipecac.)

Etoposide; Vepeside

Podophyllum peltatum (Berberidaceae) May apple, or American mandrake as it is sometimes called, grows in southeastern United States. This is a semisynthetic drug derived from the roots of May apple. In the 1980s it received approval for use as an antitumor agent in testicular and small cell lung cancer. The drug is now derived primarily from *Phexandrum* from the Himalayas, but it is now listed in CITES (Convention in Trade in Endangered Species), so commercial harvesting to derive the drug's precursor may have to return to the U.S. species. Sales of etoposide in 1990 by Bristol Myers-Squibb were more than $100 million (Duke, 1992. Personal communication). (See podophyllotoxin below.)

Hydrastine

Hydrastis canadensis (Ranunculaceae) The root of this herb, commonly referred to as goldenseal or simply Hydrastis, was a favored remedy of the Cherokee Indians in the southeastern United States where it is native. The root contains the alkaloids hydrastine, berberine, and to a lesser extent canadine, and was employed internally and externally for its wound-healing properties. The root and its extracts were used in eclectic medicine as a uterine tonic, astringent, and hemostatic. Because of its astringent action on inflamed mucous membranes, it was formerly the primary ingredient in eyewashes (Tyler et al., 1988). The bitter root was used as an ingredient in stomach bitters and tonics. It is currently a popular herb in folk medicine and is taken as a remedy, along with other herbs (e.g., garlic, cayenne pepper, and echinacea) for catarrhal conditions associated with colds and flus. There has been little modern research on this herb; most research is focusing on the alkaloid berberine, which is also found in several other North American plant genera (e.g., *Berberis*, *Mahonia*). Berberine has recognized bitter stomachic, antibacterial, antimalarial, and antipyretic activity (Merck, 1976). Hydrastic root was official in the USP in 1830, then again from 1860 to 1920. Afterward the alkaloid hydrastine and its salt hydrastine hydrochloride were official.

Ipecac

Cephaelis ipecacuanha (Rubiaceae of Madder family) Popularly known as ipecac, this is the root from a plant native to Bolivia and Brazil. Emetine is the active isoquinoline alkaloid that has amoebicide and emetic activity (Morton, 1977). It was first introduced into European medicine for diarrhea and dysentery in late 1600s. Emetine was first isolated by pharmacist-chemist Joseph Pelletier in 1817 in collaboration with Fr. Magendie. An emetine-free extract was marketed in the late 1800s as a remedy for acute dysentery, whereby the symptoms of nausea and emesis were avoided (Lloyd, 1987). Ipecac gained a reputation as "the most valuable of the vegetable emetics" and was also used as an anti-emetic and expectorant. Ipecac is one of the few drugs remaining in the USP from the first edition (1820) until the present. In the hydrochloride form, it is injected (to avoid nausea and vomiting) for its antiprotozoan properties in cases of dysentery and related amebic diseases (Tyler et al.). Presently, syrup of ipecac is widely recommended as a household first aid treatment to produce emesis in cases of various types of poisoning.

Lobeline

Lobelia inflata (Campanulaceae) Lobelia is a small annual herb native to eastern and central North America. Its primary use in folk medicine was as an expectorant and emetic, as well as convulsant, diaphoretic, expectorant, nauseant, and sedative (Duke, 1985). It was used by Indians as a substitute for tobacco, hence its name Indian tobacco. The piperidine alkaloid lobeline derived from its leaves is chemically similar to nicotine and produces similar but weaker pharmacologic effects to those of nictone on the peripheral circulation and central nervous system (CNS) (Tyler et al., 1988). The herb formerly was used in some cough preparations (Leung, 1980). Lobeline sulfate is approved as an OTC drug ingredient in lozenge form as a smoking deterrent. Lobelia was official in the USP from 1820 to 1920.

Papaine

Carica papaya (Caricaceae) Papaine is a mixture of active proteolytic enzymes from the latex of unripe fruit of the papaya, a tree native to southern Mexico, Central America, and northern South America. Traditionally, it was used as a digestant and for a host of folk medicine applications (Morton, 1977). It has been used as a meat tenderizer. One of its most recent approved uses (chymopapaine) is by neurosurgeons and orthopedic surgeons for spinal injection to shrink ruptured or slipped discs and to overcome pain from pinched spinal nerves (Morton, 1977). According to Tyler et al. (1988) "the rationale for oral or parenteral use of proteolytic enzymes in treatment of traumatically induced inflammation and edema of soft tissues is questionable" as the evidence of such utility is solely based on subjective interpretation. Papain has been listed in the USP from 1985 through the present.

Pilocarpine

Pilocarpus jaborandi (Rutaceae) This plant, traditionally known as jaborandi is native to Brazil. The imidazole alkaloid pilocarpine is a parasympathomimetic and is derived from the leaves. Pilocarpine is used topically for glaucoma (Tyler et al., 1988) acting on cholinergic receptor sites, thus mimicking the action of acetylcholine and thereby reducing intraocular pressure. Also it is used as an antidote for atropine, and stimulates secretions of the respiratory tract as well as gastric, lacrimeal, salivary, and other glands (Duke, 1985). Solutions are used in oral swabs in hospitals to stimulate salivation. The leaves were official in the USP from 1880 through the 1910 edition; the alkaloid pilocarpine is now officially recognized.

Podophyllotoxin

Podophyllum peltatum (Berberidaceae) This is a lignan from the May apple root, sometimes called American mandrake. It has a caustic action and has been used for certain papillomas (Der Marderosian and Liberti, 1988). The herb is native to southeastern Canada and the eastern United States. According to Morton the root was used by Cherokees as an emetic and purgative. It was adopted by settlers, and the crude drug was in the first edition of the USP in 1820. Later, according to Morton (1977) citing King's American Eclectic Dispensatory (1855), the extracted, powdered podophyllin was "employed as a vermifuge, treatment for constipation, typhoid fever, cholera infantum, jaundice, dysentery, chronic hepatitis, scrofula, rheumatism, dysmenorrhea, amenorrhea, kidney and bladder and prostate problems, and was employed in the treatment of gonorrhea and syphilis in place of mercurials and without their deleterious effects." Podophyllum resin has been used in modern practice as a cathartic. It was a common ingredient in over-the-counter "liver pills." The caustic resin has been used to remove skin warts, plantars warts, and papillomas of dogs, but is injurious to normal tissue, which must be protected. Ointments containing podophyllin are sometimes applied to hyperkeratotic and hypertrophic lesions (Morton, 1977). Podophyllin has been shown ineffective and unsafe for skin cancers. The drug was official from 1820 to the 1930 edition of USP, and then again from 1955 to the present.

Protoveratrines A and B

Veratrum viride (Liliaceae) Derived from American false hellebore, these drugs are antihypertensives. The plant is native to eastern and western North America. *V viride* is similar but distinctly different from European hellebore, *V album*. In the eighteenth and nineteenth centuries the powdered rhizome was employed as an analgesic used in painful diseases, epilepsy, and convulsions, pneumonia, peritonitis, and as a cardiac sedative, and in small doses to stimulate appetite (Morton, 1977). Because of toxicity, its use declined in the 1950s when its hypotensive activity was investigated, and, owing to improved chemical techniques and safety, it was administered in the form of an alkaloidal mixture, sometimes with *Rauwolfia serpentina* alkaloids (source of reserpine). Protoveratrines reduce both systolic and diastolic pressure, slow heart rate, and stimulate peripheral circulation to kidneys, liver, and extremities. Given intravenously they lower cerebral arterial resistance (Morton, 1977). "These veratrum drugs can be safely administered only in small doses. In chronic cases, tolerance develops, and, with increased dosage, there is the risk of emesis and other undesirable side-effects. Once again, enthusiasm for veratrum therapy is diminishing except in special emergencies such as hypertensive toxemia during pregnancy and the pulmonary edema which arises in acute hypertensive crises" (Morton, 1977). The crude plant and extract were official in the USP from 1820 to 1930.

Quinidine

Cinchona ledgeriana and related species (Rubiaceae) Quinidine is a quinoline alkaloid from the cinchona tree. (For information on this tree, see quinine below.) Quinidine is the stereoisomer of quinine found in the cinchona bark. It depresses myocardial excitability, conduction velocity, and to a lesser extent, contractility, and is used for cardiac arrhythmias, tachycardia, and atrial flutter and fibrillations (Tyler et al., 1988).

Quinine

(*Cinchona ledgeriana* and related species) (Rubiaceae) Quinine is a quinoline alkaloid derived from the Incan name for the Cinchona tree, *quina*, native to higher altitudes of South America. The tree was also called fever tree. It was named by the Spanish botanist Linnaeus after the legend of the Countess of Chinchon, wife of the Spanish Viceroy in the 1630s, who was saved from a malarial death when she was given doses of the bark. According to legend, she is credited with introducing the medicine to Spain and Italy (Taylor, 1945). Quinine is famous for its antimalarial and antipyretic actions and is the flavoring agent used in "tonic" water. It also has a skeletal muscle relaxing effect and is useful in prevention and treatment of nocturnal leg cramps (Tyler et al., 1988) Cinchona bark was official in the USP from 1820 to 1930. Quinine salts are still listed.

Sapogenins

Agave sisalana (Agavaceae) Sapogenins are a class of plant-derived compounds from a variety of New World plants, including plants in the monocotyledonous genera *Agave* (which includes sisal), *Dioscorea* (Mexican wild yam), and *Smilax* (sarsaparilla) (Tyler et al., 1988). For more on sapogenins, see Diosgenin above.

Sanguinarine

Sanguinaria canadensis (Papaveraceae) Bloodroot was widely used by Native Americans of eastern United States and Canada as an expectorant and strong but potentially dangerous emetic (Moerman, 1986; Vogel, 1970). It has enjoyed some folk medicine use as an escharotic for skin cancers. The isoquinoline alkaloid sanguinarine currently is used in some oral hygiene products as a dental plaque inhibitor. Bloodroot was official in the USP from 1820 through 1910.

Sarsaparilla

Smilax officinalis (Smilacaceae) This woody vine grows in Jamaica and the Caribbean, Mexico, Honduras, and northern South America. The root was employed by

New World natives for its general tonic effects and was first introduced into European medicine from Mexico in 1536, where it developed a strong following as a cure for syphilis and rheumatic conditions. It eventually developed a reputation as "blood purifier" and was official in the USP from 1820 to 1910 (Lloyd, 1929; Hobbs, 1988).

Tyler (1987) notes that sarsaparilla contains saponins that have a strong diuretic action as well as some diaphoretic, expectorant, and laxative properties. Leung (1980) cites a Chinese reference where a related Chinese species was found to be 90% effective in (presumably single-blind) clinical trials for syphilis. Although its use as a medicine declined in the early 1900s, it became a popular ingredient in a soft drink and still is used as a flavoring agent in beverages, enjoying generally regarded as safe status.

Saw Palmetto

Serenoa repens (Palmaceae) The berries of this small palm tree, which grows from South Carolina to Florida and west to Texas, have been used by Native Americans as a food and were employed in nineteenth and early twentieth century eclectic medicine as a specific for male genitourinary complaints, including irritation and swelling of the prostate (Felter and Lloyd, 1898). A liposterolic extract of the berries is approved in Germany for benign prostatic hypertrophy. Clinical studies indicate that the berry extract of *Saw palmetto* reduces frequency of urination and amount of retained urine. The berries were official in the USP from 1820 through the 1940 edition.

Storax Balsam

Liquidambar styraciflua (Hamamelidaceae) Known commonly as sweet gum, the drug derives from the resin of this tree native to the eastern United States and southern Mexico to Nicaragua. The resin was formerly used in treatment of diarrhea and dysentery. The aromatic balsam occurs in abundance only in Central American trees (Morton, 1977) and was used in pharmacy as an ingredient in compound benzoin tincture. Storax was used as a stimulant, expectorant, and antiseptic (Tyler et al., 1988). Storax was official in the USP from 1840 to 1990.

Taxol

Taxus brevifolia (Taxaceae) This new drug is receiving considerable publicity for its promising results in ovarian and breast cancers. It is derived from the bark of the Pacific yew tree, a native conifer growing under the forest canopy in the Pacific Northwest. Recent research indicates that a semisynthetic taxol can be derived from renewable quantities of European and Asian *Taxus* leaves. The drug is currently in Phase II clinical trials.

Theobromine

Theobroma cacao (Sterculiaceae) Theobromine is a xanthine alkaloid derived from the dried ripe seed of the cacao plant. It is native to Mexico and Central America. The drug is a diuretic and a smooth muscle relaxant and vasodilator, with little CNS-stimulating activity. It is thus preferred over caffeine for the treatment of cardiac edema and angina pectoris (Tyler et al.; 1988). Theobromine was official in the USP from 1860 to 1975.

Tubocurarine

Chondrodendron tomentosum (Menispermaceae) No paper on drugs from the New World would be complete without mention of this drug, an isoquinoline alkaloid, derived from Amazonian natives' use as an arrow tip poison, sometimes referred to generically as "curare." The drug is made from the intensely bitter root of a vine native to Brazil, Peru, Colombia, and Panama (Morton; 1977). The drug was introduced in 1942 as a skeletal muscle relaxant to secure muscle relaxation in surgery without deep anesthesia, to control convulsions of strychnine poisoning and tetanus, as an adjunct to shock therapy, and as a diagnostic aid in myasthenia gravis (Hein, 1984; Taylor et al., 1988). The crude drug was official in the USP from 1840 to 1900.

Turpentine

Pinus palustris, longleaf pine and *P elliottii*, slash pine (Pinaceae) Turpentine would seem more well known for its use in paint industry, but it also has had an important role in pharmacy as a rubefacient. Both pine species from which it is derived are native to southeastern United States (Morton, 1977). It formerly was used internally for treatment of gonorrhea, leucorrhea, and urinary diseases, catarrh, rheumatism, and chronic inflammation of bowels. Externally, turpentine and rosin (colophony) were employed as rubefacients and stimulants in for rheumatic and chest complaints (Morton). Terpin hydrate is the primary synthetic product from turpentine used in pharmaceuticals. The *cis*-form is used as an expectorant and also is used in veterinary medicine for treating chronic bronchitis in horses, cattle, and dogs (Morton). Pine oil, tar, and balsam listed were listed in the USP from 1820 to 1940 and then from 1970 to 1985.

Wintergreen

Gaultheria procumbens (Ericaceae) Also commonly called teaberry, 90% of the oil consists of methyl salicylate. They are considered interchangeable in pharmacy, with little distinction being made between the natural essential oil from the leaves of this eastern North American native herb. Wintergreen/methyl salicylate is also considered the same as oil of sweet birch, an essential oil distilled from the bark of the North American tree sweet birch (*Betula lenta*). The oil has rubefacient (local irritant), antiseptic and antirheumatic properties and is a common ingredient in OTC topical analgesic preparations. It is also a popular flavor in candles, chewing gums, and pharmaceutical preparations, although large doses can be toxic (Tyler et al., 1988). Various forms of wintergreen were official in the USP from 1820 to 1900. Methyl salicylate is still listed.

Witch Hazel

Hamamelis virginiana (Hamamelidaceae) The leaves, twigs, and bark of this tree native to eastern half of the United States were used by Native Americans and colonists primarily for their astringent and hemostatic properties in cases of diarrhea, eye and skin irritations, insect bites, etc. (Leung, 1980). The primary activity derives from tannins, which do not carry over into preparations during distillation. Nevertheless, the products with witch hazel are widely used for the so-called astringent properties (Tyler et al.). Witch hazel is Food and Drug Administration approved for OTC drugs for astringency in preparations such as suppositories, ointments, and lotions for treatment of hemorrhoids, itching irritation, and minor pains. Witch hazel water is the most commonly used form (Leung, 1980). Witch hazel bark was official in the USP from 1880 through 1910.

SUMMARY

The author hopes this brief review of most of the major (as well as a few minor) medicines derived from New World plants will stimulate physicians, pharmacists, and other health professionals into developing a new appreciation that the role medicinal plants have and still do play in medicine and pharmacy. As this review indicates, the development of modern medicine and pharmacy owes a great deal to these plants and plant-derived drugs. New medicinals await discovery both in the mucin-touted rain forests of Latin America and in the more temperate regions of North America, including not only the eastern forests in Appalachia but also the arid lands of the west.

A number of formerly official medicinal plants are still used by a growing number of American consumers for minor complaints and as well as for prophylaxis. A case in point is the widespread use of the herb Echinacea (*Echinacea purpurea; E angustifolia*), sometimes referred to as purple coneflower. Echinacea root was one of the most widely used medicines employed by Indians of the Great Plains. The plant caught the attention of a German pharmacist Dr. Gerard Madaus, who in the late 1930s imported some to Germany for research purposes. Madaus eventually found a significant level of immunostimulant activity in the leaf and root extracts of echinacea, which has been confirmed by other researchers. Presently in Germany, extracts of both Echinacea leaf and root are officially approved by the Ministry of Health as medicines for colds, flus, certain inflammations, and as "immunostimulants," with no reports of any adverse reactions (Foster, 1991). Echinacea is one of the most popular herbs in use by consumers, herbalists, and holistic physicians in the United States. What other promising plants from our own hemisphere have we possibly overlooked?

Unfortunately, there exist significant regulatory and patent roadblocks to the approval of many "soft drugs" that formerly have been official plant medicines. With the present cost of a new drug application approaching $231 million, pharmaceutical companies simply do not have economic incentives to research many traditionally used herbs and medicinal plants unless patent protection is available. In the case of most herbals, they are simply not patentable. Despite their documentation of safety and efficacy (historically and in modern scientific studies usually conducted in Europe or Asia), many of these natural products, formerly used in crude drug or extract form, cannot find an appropriate regulatory standard for approval in self-medication in the United States. Some experts have suggested development of a new regulatory category for some of these medicines. (Tyler, 1992a,b).

Although no one could responsibly suggest that all herbs and medicinal plants that were formerly official should be approved for OTC sale merely on the basis of their previous use, some pharmacy experts have indeed called for the development of regulatory reform in the United States in which certain herbs and medicinal plants that enjoyed former official status once again be allowed sold in the marketplace with reasonable health and therapeutic claims, as long as new scientific data do not show them to be either unsafe or ineffective (Tyler, 1992b).

Just as Columbus unwittingly discovered a new treasure trove of culinary and medicinal plants in the New World of the fifteenth century, plants of the Western Hemisphere will continue to provide valuable new medicines for a variety of health care applications into the twenty-first century.

BIBLIOGRAPHY

Anon. "What to dispense?" Pharmacy History 34:48,

Blumenthal M. Focus on rain forest medicinals. HerbalGram 27:8–10, 1992.

Boyl W. Official Herbs: Botanical Substances in the United States Pharmacopoeias 1820–1990. East Palestine, OH: Buckeye Naturopathic Press, 1991.

British Herbal Pharmacopoeia. 1983. British Herbal Medicine Association.

Der Marderosian A, Liberti LE. Natural Products Medicine: A Scientific Guide to Foods, Drugs, Cosmetics. Philadelphia, PA: Geo. F. Stickley Co., 1988.

Der Marderosian A, Yelvigi MS. Medicine and drugs in colonial America. Am J Pharmacy July/August, 1976, pp. 113–120.

Reprinted with permission as Classic Botanical Reprint 222, American Botanical Council, Austin, TX.

Duke JA. CRC Handbook of Medicinal Herbs. Boca Raton, FL: CRC Press, 1985.

Elisabetsky E. The pharmacopeia from the forest. Garden Nov/Dec 4–6, 1990.

Elks J, Ganellin CR. Dictionary of Drugs: Chemical Data, Structures and Bibliographies. New York: Chapman and Hall, Scientific Data Division, 1990.

Farnsworth NR, Akerele O, Bingel AS, Soejarto DD, Guo ZG. Medicinal plants in therapy. Bull World Health Organ 63:965–981, 1985. Reprinted with permission by American Botanical Council, Austin, TX, Classic Botanical Reprint 212.

Felter HW, Lloyd JU. King's American Dispensatory. Portland, OR: Eclectic Medical Publications, 1983.

Foster S. Echinacea: Nature's Immune Herb. Rochester, VT: Healing Arts Press, 1991.

Foster S. The Badianus manuscript: The first herbal from the Americas. HerbalGram 27:12–17, 1992.

Foster S, Duke JA. 1990. Peterson's Field Guide to Eastern and Central Medicinal Plants. Boston, MA: Houghton-Mifflin, 1990.

Glasby JS. Dictionary of Plants Containing Secondary Metabolites. New York: Taylor & Francis, 1991.

Griffenhagen GB. The materia medica of Christopher Columbus. Pharmacy History 34:131–145, 1992.

Hein WH. The history of curare research. In: Hein W-H. Botanical Drugs of the Americas in the Old and New Worlds. Stuttgart: Wissenschaftliche Verlagsgesellschaft, 1984.

Hobbs C. Sarsaparilla: A literature review. HerbalGram 17, 1988.

King, SR. Conservation and tropical medicinal plant research. HerbalGram 27:28–35, 1992.

Kingsbury J. Columbus as a botanist. Cornell Plantations Vol:000–000, 1990.

Krieg MB. Green Medicine: The Search for Plants that Heal. New York: Rand McNally, 1964.

Leung AY. Encyclopedia of Common Ingredients Used in Foods, Drugs and Cosmetics. New York: John Wiley and Sons, 1980.

Lewis W, Elvin-Lewis M. Medical Botany: Plants Affecting Man's Health. New York: John Wiley and Sons, 1977.

Lloyd JU. Cephalis ipecacuanha. Pamphlet reprinted from The Western Druggist.

Lloyd JU. Origin and History of all the Pharmacopeial Vegetable Drugs. Cincinnati, OH: Caxton Press, 1929.

Martindale W. The Extra Pharmacopoeia, 22nd ed. London: The Pharmaceutical Press, 1944.

Merck Index, 9th ed. Rahway, NJ: Merck & Co., 1976.

Millspaugh CF. American Medicinal Plants. New York: Dover Publications, 1974.

Moerman DE. Medicinal Plants of Native America. 2 Vols. Research Reports in Ethnobotany, Contribution 2; Technical Reports, 19. Ann Arbor, MI: University of Michigan Museum of Anthropology, 1986.

Morton JF. Major Medicinal Plants: Botany, Culture and Uses. Springfield, IL: Charles C. Thomas, 1977.

Risse GB. Transcending cultural barriers: The European reception of medicinal plants from the Americas. In Hein W-H. Botanical Drugs of the Americas in the Old and New Worlds. Stuttgart: Wissenschaftliche Verlagsgesellschaft, 1984.

Schultes RE. Dwindling forest: medicinal plants of the Amazon. Harvard Med Alum Bull Vol. 65: 1991.

Schultes RE, Raffauf RF. Healing Forest: Medicinal and Toxic Plants of the Northwest Amazon. Portland, OR: Dioscorides Press, 1991.

Taylor N. Cinchona in Java: The Story of Quinine. New York: Greenberg Publisher, 1945.

Tyler VE. Plant drugs in the 21st century. Economic Botany 40:2790–288, reprinted with permission as Classic Botanical Reprint 207, American Botanical Council, Austin, TX, 1986.

Tyler VE. The New Honest Herbal. Philadelphia: George F. Stickley Co., 1987.

Tyler VE, Brady LR, Robbers JE. Pharmacognosy, 9th ed. Philadelphia, PA: Lea & Febiger, 1988.

Tyler VE. 1992a. Natural products and medicine: an overview. Presented at "Tropical Forest Medical Resources and the Conservation of Biodiversity" sponsored by the Rainforest Alliance's Periwinkle Project and the New York Botanical Garden's Institute of Economic Botany, The Rockefeller University, New York, January 1992.

Tyler, VE. 1992b. Phytomedicines in Western Europe: their potential impact on herbal medicine in the United States. Presented at "Human Medicinal Agents from Plants," American Chemical Society 203d National Meeting, San Francisco, CA, April 5–10, 1992.

Uphof JC Th. Dictionary of Economic Plants. 2d ed. Lehre, Germany: Verlag Von J. Cramer, 1968.

Viola HJ, Margolis C. Seeds of Change: A Quintecentennial Commemoration. Washington, DC: Smithsonian Institution, 1991.

Vogel VJ. American Indian Medicine. Norman, OK: University of Oklahoma Press, 1970. □

Chapter 10

European Animal Diseases Brought to the New World

R. Allen Packer, D.V.M., Ph.D.

ABSTRACT

Beginning with Columbus' second voyage to the New World in 1493, domesticated animals have been imported to establish herds and flocks for the development of animal agriculture and as mounts for the early explorers. Some of these imports harbored agents of disease that were transmitted to healthy animals during their ocean voyage or to their offspring born in the New World. Some of these diseases were eradicated, others have persisted to the present.

The entry of explorers into the New World in 1492 was soon followed by importation of domesticated animals. In 1493, Columbus commanded 17 ships that carried seeds, plants, trees and a number of animals. Those included were a bull, several cows, a horse, eight pigs, goats, and very probably some chickens. There are no records as to the fate of these animals, but the pigs "landed running," found the living conditions very favorable, and rapidly increased in number. Other Spanish explorers brought pigs to accompany the troops as a mobile meat supply; however, some became feral living and prospering in the woods.

Additional early importations of record include these examples:

1527 horses to Florida
1538 horses and pigs to Florida
1553 cattle and pigs to Nova Scotia
1604 cattle, horses and pigs to Arcadia

From Microbiology, Immunology and Preventive Medicine. College of Veterinary Medicine, Iowa State University, Ames, Iowa

1609 sheep to Jamestown, Virginia
1620 goats, pigs and chickens to Plymouth, Massachusetts.

These early imports started herds and flocks that provided food for colonists and, as numbers increased, opened an export market for meat products.

Importation of animals has continued from these early times to the present day. Through the years, as animal agriculture developed, importations from Great Britain and Western Europe have consisted of breeding stock for the purpose of introducing desirable traits in offspring. Beginning in the last half of the 1800s, breeders in Britain and continental Europe were more advanced in the selection and breeding of animals possessing certain desirable characteristics, such as feed efficiency and carcasses having less fat.

Considering the frequency of "carriers" among all animal populations or those animals suffering some sickness on arrival in the United States, each animal imported could be a potential spreader of disease. In the early days when there were no quarantine or inspection requirements for imports, many diseases were introduced that spread among the native livestock, costing large sums of money to control or to eradicate.

The ability to distinguish one disease from another is essential in tracing their origins, following their spread, and in the application of effective control measures. Some infectious diseases are clinically quite distinct and were described in ancient times. For example, Aristotle, 350 B.C. described a disease of cattle that most certainly was contagious pleuropneumonia. The French veterinarian, Bourgelat, gave the first complete description of this disease in 1769. At this time the disease had spread over all Europe, taking a heavy toll. Nevertheless, the ability to recognize the disease eventually led to its control.

Bovine pleuropneumonia was first introduced into

the United States in 1843 by an infected dairy cow unloaded at Long Island, New York, from the Netherlands. The disease spread widely in the eastern states and extended to the west. As a result, cattlemen became alarmed and began measures to control the disease. Federal and state governments appropriated funds to that end. In 1884 an agency under the US Department of Agriculture, the Bureau of Animal Industry (BAI) was established. It was staffed with veterinarians and other specialists and charged with the eradication of bovine pleuropneumonia. Eight years later, 1892, the United States was declared free of the disease, and it has remained free. The "stamping-out" method, that is, slaughter and burial of the infected and exposed, so successful in eliminating pleuropneumonia established a procedure for the eradication of other infectious diseases of animals.

Other diseases imported from Europe and subsequently eradicated are:

Foot-and-mouth disease (restricted to cloven-hoofed species.) 9 outbreaks, 1879–1929.
Fowl pest (domestic fowl) 1929
Glanders (equine, man) 1934
Dourine (equine) 1942
Exotic Newcastle (poultry) 1974
Hog cholera (swine only) 1978 (origin in doubt)

The cost of eradication of the foot-and-mouth disease outbreak of 1914 was $9,000,000. During the 1924 epizootic that occurred in California, the numbers of animals slaughtered and buried were 49,781 cattle; 24,978 sheep; 20,988 swine; and 808 goats. In addition some 45,000 deer were slaughtered to contain the outbreak.

Examples of infectious diseases from Europe that have persisted and spread are bovine tuberculosis; pseudorabies—swine, cattle; rabies—canine strain, canine distemper, equine contagious metritis, strangles (equine); marek's disease—chickens; scrapie—sheep, and bovine brucellosis.

Federally funded programs have sharply reduced the incidence of some of these diseases (tuberculosis and brucellosis), but they have not yet been eradicated. A number of other disease agents including those of mange, scabies, and internal parasitism also have accompanied imports to the New World.

REFERENCES

Bierer BW. History of animal plagues of North America. Reprinted by Washington, DC: US Department of Agriculture, 1940.

Graves W, ed. Spain in the Americas. Washington, DC: National Geographic Magazine. February 1992.

Law J. Lung plague of cattle. In: Law J, ed, Textbook of Veterinary Medicine, Vol IV. Ithaca, NY: 1902, pp. 598–623.

Towne CW, Wentworth EN. Pigs from caves to cornbelt. Norman, OK: University of Oklahoma Press. 1950.

US Animal Health Association. Foreign Animal Diseases. Richmond, VA: 1984.

Wiser V, Mark LM, Purchase HG, eds. 100 years of Animal Health, 1884–1984. Beltsville, MD: The Associates of The National Agricultural Library, 1987.

Chapter 11

Contribution of the New World Food to the World Supply

Michel Fondu* and Jean-Claude Dillon[†]

The "discovery" of the new world by Christopher Columbus brought Europeans in contact with new food. Their alphabetic classification gives the following: avocado, beans (lima-kidney), cacao, cashew, chili, maize (corn), muscovy duck, papaya, peanuts, pecan, pineapple, pumpkin, squash, sunflower, sweet potato, tomato, turkey, vanilla, and white potato.

This classification is not very useful, and if we want to consider the importance those foodstuffs have taken in other parts of the world, we have to use other criteria: nutritional value and gastronomical properties.

In a period where the level of life of the large majority of European population was rather low (and still is in some regions), new food sources were of interest as far as they could enhance the nutritive value of the diet, be easier to cultivate, replace a food more difficult to get, ameliorate the organoleptic characteristic (taste, color) of the plates, or introduce new pleasant types of foodstuffs (cacao).

Based on these criteria, the following classification can be proposed:

For their nutritive value: white potato, maize (corn), sunflower, peanuts, papaya, and sweet potato.

For their organoleptic or folkloric character: Tomatoes give color and taste to meals; is it possible to imagine the Italian gastronomy without tomatoes? Turkey meat was not used frequently till a few years ago. However, what would Christmas have been in Great Britain without the traditional turkey? Cacao and all its derivatives; and Vanilla.

And the rest of the list: those foodstuffs eaten from

* Scientific Director, ILSI Europe, Av. Mounier, 83, B-1200 Brussels, Belgium
† Institut National Agronomique, Chaire de Nutrition Humaine, Rue C. Bernard, 16, F-75005 Paris, France

time to time such as avocado, lima and kidney beans, cashew, pecan, pumpkin, and squash but, till now, had no important impact on our food habits.

"Till now" means that, until the last 20 years, our food habits were not easy to change and that for most of those new foods, time was needed before their value was understood and recognized.

It is not easy to follow the path of the potato (white potato) in Europe. They had different names from country to country. Even in the same country, the product was known in one region and not in another. In fact, the ways botanists informed each other on this new crop were more linked to personal relationship than to logical, geographical approaches. We do not speak about an economical interest, which was then nonexistent. But there are two more difficulties. To our knowledge, no attempt has been made until now to produce a global historical review on the penetration of this crop into Europe, the U.K. included. In the beginning, the denominations "sweet" and "white" potato were used indistinctly for both crops. In Haiti, the sweet potato was called batata. And between batata, patata, and potato, the difference is small. The Italians called it tartuffoli, from the Italian tartuffo (truffle); tartuffoli (small truffle). And between tartuffoli and kartoffel in German, the difference is also small. We may add that tartoufle was the first name given to the potato in French.

What seems certain is that the first reproduction of the potato was done by a Flemish botanist Carolus Clausius in 1588 (water colors in Plantin Moretus Museum-Antwerp-Belgium).

How did he get the crop? Probably as follows: in 1565, Philip II, King of Spain, sent potatoes to Pope Pius IV and one of the Pope's assistants (collaborators) sent two crops to the Governor of Mons, Belgium, Philippe de Sivry, who dispatched them to Carolus Clausius.[1] The botanist John Gerard (England) received some seeds from Carolus Clausius and described them in his "Herbae" (1596) as bastard potato or *papus arbiculatus*. The same year the Swiss botanist Gaspard Bauhin (1560–1624) gave it the botanical name, *Solanum Tuberosum-Esculantum*.

There is, however, a difference between an interest shown by botanists and use as foodstuff by the common people.

As William H. McNeill wrote,[2] "why should farmers give up familiar routines and crop rotations to make room for strange plants that looked very different from what they already knew, and required rather strenuous cultivation during the growing season to keep down weeds? Why start eating something unfamiliar that might be poisonous and that had to be prepared differently from the foods already tried, tested, and available?" Those persons who have to cope with hunger in the world know this point is still a very difficult one to solve.

As long as familiar foods were available in suitable quantity, and enough land was accessible for cultivating established crops in traditional ways, farmers had little or no incentive to experiment with anything as strange and risky as this New World crop often, in practice, turned out to be.

For that reason change came slowly, especially in France where the first description was done in 1614. In 1698, an English medical doctor (Lister) was surprised when visiting France not to find potatoes. When consulting French cookery documents of this period or books describing the way of life during the 17th century, it is not easy even to find the word potato.[3] Food scarcity was needed to modify this situation.

However, it was quite different in other countries. The book "Ouverture de Cuisine,"[4] for instance, had been published in 1604 by Lancelot de Casteau, who was chief cook of the Prince Bishop of Liège (Belgium). In it, amid the list of plants and herbs to be used, "tartoufle" and chestnuts can be found. A number of methods of preparation are described: boiled tartoufles; tartoufles baked in fire like chestnuts; slices cooked in butter, indicating that at least for the rich people, tartoufles were part of the normal culinary uses.

With regard to Britain, the new root destined to make the greatest impact on British eating habits was, of course, the potato.[5] Sir Francis Drake brought some roots to England, having apparently obtained them at Cartagena in Colombia. But on his homeward journey, he touched the Virginian coast to pick up some English settlers; and this led to a misunderstanding about the provenance of the first English potatoes. For many years afterward they were called "Virginia" potatoes to distinguish them from the sweet or "Spanish" variety. Their introduction into Ireland, ascribed variously to Sir Walter Raleigh and the looting of ships' stores from a wrecked Armada vessel (Spanish), probably took place no later than 1588.

It was a long time before Virginia potatoes became at all common in England. Through most of the 17th century it is clear from recipes they were regarded as a specialty food, whether baked in pies or used to garnish rick boiled meats, such as beef olives, turkeys, capons, chickens, and game birds.

In most cases, sweet or Virginia potatoes could be used interchangeably, and probably were, because sweet potatoes continued to be as well or even better liked than the Virginian ones. It was late in the century before the starch potential of the latter was recognized and boiled, mashed potatoes came into occasional use as a foundation for pudding, in place of bread or cereal flour.

In Ireland, however, the native population was quick to appreciate the virtues of the new roots. Not only were they easier to grow than oats and barley, they were also safer. It was an area of turbulence and uprisings, with the military practicing a scorched-earth policy. An underground crop of potatoes was much more difficult to find and destroy than a visible one of standing corn.

Before 1617 soldiers who returned to England reported whole fields in Ireland overrun by potatoes. Irish influence, no doubt, accounted for the cultivation of potatoes in Lancashire. Here, as in Ireland, oats were the common cereals, and potatoes were received more readily by oat bread eaters than they were in wheaten bread areas. This is confirmed by the fact that in English 18th century cookery book[6] potatoes are used in cheap soup but not in potable soup, charitable soup which may be used at any gentleman's table, veal gravy soup, beef gravy soup.

Potatoes, which had been cultivated in Belgium since 1680, were exported to the United Kingdom between 1763 and 1773.[7] In England, they were increasingly cultivated in the second half of the century, because each time there was a poor cereal harvest, potatoes advanced in popularity. As mentioned, at first potatoes were grown only in gardens, but later, they were developed as a field crop.

Those examples illustrate that it is very difficult to generalize the idea that although potatoes were an important source of calories and vitamin C, they were quickly considered as being a good replacer of existing food. Even when, like the potato, the plant can adapt to poor soil and different climatic conditions, the production per acre is high and the storage rather easy.

Nevertheless, by the late 17th and 18th centuries, the American domestications were being assimilated with increasing speed to global farming and culinary patterns. This is not the sole reason for the population explosion of the past two centuries, however, it is one of the major factors of this growth.

Although the intake of potatoes has been decreasing since the end of the World War II, potato and maize are still two of the four chief staples of the human diet.

The history of maize is much more difficult to follow. It came to Europe and later to other continents, and found its place where the climatic conditions favored its production. It did well in mountain valleys from Spain to the Balkans, it also prospered in the Po valley (Italy) and in the Danube plains. In the beginning it was used without the knowledge of ways to prepare it, and a population having learned to live on cornmeal mush began to suffer from pellagra.

On the same continent and in Rhodesia, Africa, the importance of maize when the first settlers arrived in 1892 cannot be determined, but the evidence available suggests that since that time, it has become of considerably greater importance as a diet item in many areas. The entire development of cash cropping based on maize appears to have taken place since the last decade of the 19th century. In a book published in 1909, Horne indicated that in 1901 a fearful cattle disease broke out on the eastern border of Southern Rhodesia. Strange although it may appear, the result of this disease was to set in motion the first real stimulus toward progress in agriculture. Old landowners collected the remainder of their cattle and, as they were not allowed to let them stray onto other ground, they set about to break up their land and put it under cultivation.

The annual report of the Department of Agriculture in 1910 suggests that maize and little else was being grown by Europeans because of the simplicity of its cultivation, the sure demand, and comparative certainty of a crop.[8]

In Africa, cassava contributes to about 40% of the calories consumed. This starchy root constitutes the second leading vegetable crop of the world (Irish potatoes are the leading one). Cassava (manioc, manihot) is native to the tropical areas of the New World between the Tropics of Cancer and Capricorn. After the discovery of America, the Portuguese took cassava to Africa and the Spanish took it to the Philippines. Later, the crop was introduced into India. During the 16th century, various colonial powers in Africa promoted extensive growing of cassava because it is drought resistant and also immune to attacks by locusts and wild animals, as the most commonly grown varieties contained poisonous cyanides (which can be removed by processing). Hence, millions of people in the tropical belt came to rely on this crop as a staple food.[9–12]

Tomatoes have been classified in the second group of foodstuffs coming from the New World because of their organoleptic characteristics: color and taste. It does not mean that they do not have nutritional properties; their content in vitamins A and C has to be taken into consideration as they have played, and still play, a role in the nutritional status in countries such as Italy and France where they are consumed in large quantities.

Tomatoes initially considered ornamental plants, were first used as foodstuffs in Italy during the 18th century and in France during the 19th century.

Regarding cacao, it is needless to stress the importance of this new food in other regions of the world: cacao also is considered in this paper a gastronomical item and the source of a large number of new food commodities. We also must remember the great economical importance of this crop for some countries.

Having rapidly reviewed what are considered the most important new crops for other parts of the world, and taking into consideration the fact that "energy and nutrients are required for meeting basic metabolic needs (including growth in children and adolescents, pregnancy and lactation in women) and physical and mental activity both for work and recreation,"[13] a question has to be raised.

Why did the introduction of those crops into Europe take such an important part in the growth of population and the economical development in Europe and not in other parts of the world, including the New World where they came from? The answer is to be found in the many factors that affect the nutritional status of new foods.

A number of underlying determinants influence the ability of individuals or households to acquire and effectively use enough good quality and safe food, and other goods and services needed for their nutritional well-being. These determinants relate to household food security, health and social services, and care and feeding practices. These factors are interrelated and may be affected by the distribution of resources and knowledge within societies and between societies. Household food security entails access to the food needed for a healthy life, adequate in terms of quality, quantity, safety, and cultural acceptance.

Access to, and utilization of, health care services including environmental health and sanitation, is a key determinant of nutritional status, and one that can be influenced by policy measures. Finally, there are basic determinants related to the historical and sociocultural background of the society, the structure and operation of the political system, its resources (land, water, and people), and external factors (macroeconomic conditions, climate).

Linked to the direct use of new crops by our population are those used as feeding stuffs. In this respect, maize can be considered of the utmost importance, perhaps as important as feed for cattle as potatoes were for human beings.

Another point to mention is the sunflower. Imported as new crop from the New World, the sunflower, which in the beginning was also considered as an ornamental plant, is now largely cultivated for its rich oil (polyunsaturated fatty acids) and used as table oil and as main component of mayonnaise and margarine. It even competes with soy-bean oil, which is still coming as seed from the "New World".

The introduction of new crops in the Old World can, in fact, be considered as providential. They helped to almost suppress food scarcity in those countries where they could be cultivated and accepted as food.

REFERENCES

1. Moulin L. Les liturgies de la table. Mercator, 1988.
2. McNeill WH. American food crops in the old world in seeds of change. *Smithsonian*, 1991.
3. Goubert P. La Vie Quotidienne des Paysans Français au 17è Siécle Hachette.
4. de Casteau L. Ouverture de Cuisine (1604). Antwerp/Bruxelles: De Schutter, 1983.
5. Wilson CA. Food and Drink in Britain. London: Constable, 1973.
6. English 18th Century Cookery. The Living Past. Ray Bloom, Ltd.
7. White LJ. Food and history. In: Food, Man and Society. Plenum Press, 1975.
8. Miracle M. Maize in Tropical Africa. Madison, WI: The University Of Wisconsin Press, 1966.
9. Hobhouse H. Seeds of Change. New York: Harper & Row, 1987.
10. Harlan JR. Crops and man-American Society of Agronomy, Madison, WI, 1975.
11. Sauer CO. Agricultural Origins and Dispersals. The American Geographical Society, New York 1952.
12. Heiser GB Jr. Seeds of Civilization. The Story of Food. Freeman, San Francisco, 3d ed., 1981.
13. Global assessment and analysis of current problems and trends in nutrition. Background draft paper prepared for the FAO/WHO International Conference on Nutrition. Rome, December 1992.   □

Chapter 12

Early Spanish Physicians and Hospitals in Cuba

Marcos A. Iglesias, M.B.A.

ABSTRACT

Very little is known about the early history of medicine in the Caribbean. Five hundred years ago medicine practitioners from Europe started to settle in the New World. Hospitals were built in very rudimentary houses to care for the sick. Diseases were received and transmitted by the new settlers. The author, a philatelist and a Columbus scholar, uses postage stamps to highlight the introduction of European medicine in Cuba.

The history of medicine in Cuba, specifically within the city of Havana from 1550 through 1799, has been recorded in the Minutes of the City Council of Havana.[1] During this period, the City Council authorized the following professionals of medicine to practice: master surgeons, surgeons or barbers, 39; Romancist surgeons (surgeons who did not speak Latin), 2; doctors in medicine, 11; licentiates in medicine, 6; practical physicians, 1; bachelors in medicine, 27; apothecaries or pharmacists, 19; midwives, 2; and protomedicos (Physicians to the King), 17.[1]

The City Council also granted the licenses of "flebotomiano" (phlebotomist, a person who could bleed), "algebraist" (a surgeon specially dedicated to treat dislocations of the bones), herbalists, and oculists. The minutes do not record any of these, but among the authorizations granted there were persons who practiced their respective "specialties."

The license to practice medicine in Havana was extended to the "Republic of Cuba" (the Minutes frequently refer to the country as "this republic," although at the time it was a Spanish colony).[1]

The degrees were granted by universities or by protomedicos. Until the University of Havana was established in 1728, Cubans opting for the degrees that would authorize them to practice medicine had to travel to the universities of Mexico City or Santo Domingo (Dominican Republic). Other options were Lima (Peru), or Spain (Alcala de Henares, Salamanca, Valladolid, Barcelona, etc.), however distances to those places were too far.

By resorting to historical data, we are able to identify and to relate some facts, inasmuch as the Cuban Postal Administration has given us very little to include in the history of medicine in Cuba.

MEDICAL DOCTORS

Physicians of that period have not been recorded on stamps. The first physicians to arrive in Cuba came with Christopher Columbus on his first voyage, one surgeon or "fisico" in each ship. Therefore, the first western doctors arrived in Cuba with Christopher Columbus when he sighted Cuba on October 27, 1492. (Fig. 1)

As with most things related to Columbus, the names of these physicians and the ships in which they sailed are confusing. The roster of the fleet includes the following: On board the Santa Maria, the flagship, was Master Alonso, Physician from Moguer. It is believed he remained in Hispaniola with the other members of the crew under Diego de Arana. Inasmuch as all were killed by the natives, he would be the first physician buried in America.

In the roster of the Pinta, Miss Alice Gould[2] mentions Maestre Diego, surgeon (sometimes referred to as "barber"). Until proved to the contrary, I am of the opinion that Maestre Diego returned to Spain on the Pinta.

The roster of the Nina also shows again some confusion. Records show that the physician aboard was

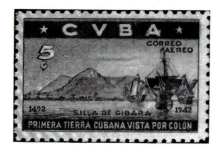

Figure 1.

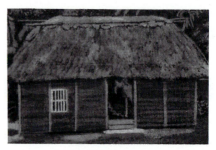

Figure 3.

Juan Sanchez (Maestre Juan, from Cordoba). There is enough evidence to believe that he was an apothecary.[3]

All three physicians left Cuba rather early: Maestre Diego in the Pinta toward the island of Babeque on 21st of November 1492, when Martin Alonso deserted Columbus. The other two left Cuba on December 5, 1492, toward the island that Columbus believed the natives called "Bohio" (Haiti).

In Cuba, the first authorization for medical practice was granted to Juan Gomez, the "Barber and Surgeon of this Village" on August 26, 1552. The last such license of this period was granted to Don Bartolome de Salas as surgeon, on January 18, 1788.

The most influential physician in Havana was Don Francisco de Teneza, from Caceres, Spain. Dr. Teneza practiced with tremendous influence his designation as physician, master surgeon, midwife, exclusive judge (juez privativo) and first protomedico, which conferred him the right to grant licenses to practice medicine.

Dr. Teneza also inspected pharmacies, kept continuous vigilance on the municipal and country authorities, claimed prebends, lands, roads, rights of way, honoraria, and many other benefits. He also used his privilege as protomedico and as member of the Inquisition of which he was a Fellow of the Holy Office.

HOSPITALS

During the same period, "The Minutes" mention the following hospitals in Havana: Saint Philip the Royal, Saint Francis of Paula, Our Lady of Bethelem, San Ambrosio, Our Lady of Pilar, Saint Lazarus, and Regla.

The Cuban Postal Administration has recorded very little about hospitals. Stamp Scott 1300[4] shows the ruins of the Saint Francis of Paula hospital (Fig. 2).

Around 1530 there was a hospital in Santiago (de Cuba). According to Irene Wright,[5] the hospital and its chapel were housed in "bohios" (huts thatched with palm leaves, similar to bohios built by the primitive inhabitants of Cuba) (Fig. 3).

By 1535, part of the petty fines (penas de camara) levied in Havana were appropriated for the support of hospitals and churches. According to documents of the time, the first hospital built in Havana probably was founded before 1545, most likely at one side of "La Fuerza" fortress (Fig. 4). The Minutes indicate that "it [the hospital] could put in danger the adjacent military fortress."[1] The construction served as church and hospital.

Dr. Angulo (not a physician), the first governor of Cuba to take permanent residence in Havana (1550), claimed to have built an addition to the hospital and to have erected two-story buildings in the back part of the building, which were to be rented to provide income for the institution.

Hospital Saint Philip the Royal (San Felipe el Real)

This hospital is recorded in the Minutes under different names. In 1597, a hospital with this name was entrusted to the congregation of Saint John of God. Therefore,

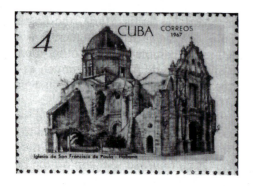

Figure 2.

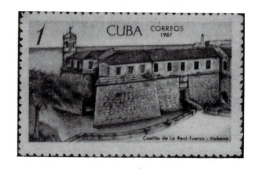

Figure 4.

74

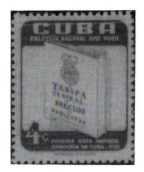

Figure 5.

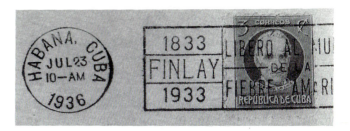

Figure 7.

the hospital is frequently referred to as Hospital Saint John of God (it was customary to name hospitals according to the religious congregation that administered them). Again, in 1603, the Minutes indicate that the Hospital Saint Philip the Royal" was given to the congregation of Saint John of God, although the construction had not been finished." The same Saint John of God Hospital appears in the records of the archives in 1692. During the occupation of Havana by England (1762), it served as headquarters to part of the British forces that occupied Havana. In other sections of the Minutes the same hospital is called "Convent Royal Hospital of Saint Philip and Saint James" and "Convent Royal Hospital of Saint John of God."[1]

Hospital Saint Francis of Paula

The San Francisco de Paula Hospital (Fig. 2) was founded on a bequest of Presbyter Don Nicolas Estebez Borges in Havana, Cuba, in 1665. Presbyter Estebez specified in his bequest that the hospital was to be built with the purpose "to heal poor women."[6]

The construction of the complex, including the hospital, a hermitage and a church, in the Campeche section of the City (so called because it was inhabited mainly by Mexican Indians brought from Campeche, Mexico, after 1564), started in 1666. This section was located near the harbor. The hospital was one of the first built in America. (In 1715 the Acts mention the Hospital of Paula, for women. This hospital was built close to the harbor and existed, with many modifications until the 20th century.)

Hospital Our Lady of Belen (or Bethelem)

This hospital, located in the Convent of Our Lady of Belen, is mentioned for the first time in 1715. That year the friars of the convent requested and obtained authorization to build an arch over the street to connect the two sections of the building to provide better sanitary conditions for the patients. The arch was built (and still exists) over the Acosta street, in Old Havana. It was a hospital for "convalescents" and for the "sanitation of the Navy."[1]

Hospital San Ambrosio

The convent of Saint Agustine was earmarked in 1762 as a Hospital for the "Troop and Royal Hospital," and was assigned to the Spanish troop. It was called Hospital San Ambrosio.

Hospital Our Lady of Pilar

This hospital was built outside the city walls, in the section of the city called Jesus Maria. It was mainly used by the slaves who inhabited that area in great numbers.

Hospital Saint Lazarus

The Saint Lazarus hospital was built outside the city walls, in the area then called Monte Vedado, near the San Lazaro inlet. The hospital was built to take care of those affected with the "disease of Saint Lazarus" (leprosy). In 1748 the King instructed the Governor of Cuba, Don Francisco Cagigal de la Vega, to look after

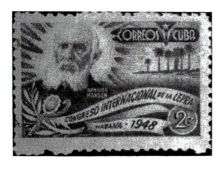

Figure 6.

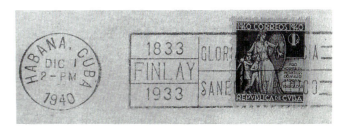

Figure 8.

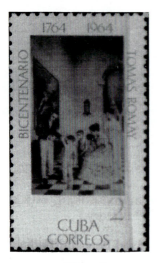

Figure 9.

the needs of the hospital. There were between 60 and 65 patients "of all colors, sex, and ages." The annual cost to operate the hospital was estimated at 3,676 pesos and 4 reales. The hospital was a complex of buildings that included the hermit, a house to lodge the attendants, and 60 "bohios" or huts. In 1749, Dr. Francisco Teneza recorded the need of 6 "arrobas" (150 pounds) of oil per annum for the lamp of the hospital.[1]

Hospital of Regla
This hospital was located in the Sanctuary of Regla, across Havana harbor, in the town of Regla. The hospital was equipped with 18 beds.

PHARMACY
The only stamp directly related to this period is Scott 582 (Fig. 5). Owing to the abuse of some pharma- cists who charged excessive prices for medicines, the "Illustrious City Council" approved a "General Tariff of Prices of Medicine" in 1723. The cover of the book is shown in the stamp. This book was the first printed in Cuba.

DISEASES
The main diseases that scourged the population were leprosy (the so called "disease of Saint Lazarus"), yellow fever (black vomit), and smallpox.

Cuba issued a stamp to commemorate the International Congress of Leprosy (S-414) held in Havana in 1948 (Fig. 6).

About yellow fever there is a whole story related to Dr. Carlos J. Finlay's discovery of the relationship between the sick person, the mosquito, and the future sick person. However, Dr. Finlay's discovery took place in the 19th century. To illustrate yellow fever philatelically, what better homage than the two cancellations "Finlay Liberated the World of Yellow Fever" (Fig. 7) and "Finlay—Glory of Science, Cleaned up the Tropic" (Fig. 8). Regarding smallpox, stamp S-928 (Fig. 9), shows Dr. Tomas Romay vaccinating his own son.

REFERENCES
1. All medical related portions of "The Minutes" have been compiled in two volumes by Dr. Jose Lopez Sanchez and published by the Ministry of Health, Havana, Cuba.
2. Alice B. Gould dedicated many years of her life to search the "Archivos de Indias," Seville, Spain.
3. George Griffenhagen, "Drugs Discovered by Christopher Columbus." Topical Time, Vol. 42, No. 2.
4. Scott Standard Postage Stamp Catalogue, 1992.
5. I. A. Wright "The Early History of Cuba 1492–1586," Octagon Books, New York, 1970.
6. Dr. Jorge Le-Roy y Cassa "Historia del hospital San Francisco de Paula," La Habana, 1958. □

Chapter 13

Spain, Portugal, Christopher Columbus, and the Jewish Physician: Introduction

Sheldon G. Cohen, M.D.

"We have just enough religion to make us hate, but-
not enough to make us love one another."
Jonathan Swift
Thoughts on Various Subjects from
Miscellanies (1711)

AUGUST 2, 1492

Whether by coincidence, design of an unknown force, or direction of fate, calendars mark the second of August 1492 as momentous in the annals of tragedy and cruelty, and also as a landmark in an epochal age of discovery. In the crossing of paths and through separate, yet interwoven, events records of this date chronicle extremes of fortune—ill for the Jews of Spain and bright for an Italian-born sailor and the Spanish fleet of three ships under his command.

On August 2, 1492, another event in the never-ending series of persecutions and upheavals befalling the Jewish people occurred in Spain. The date was particularly noteworthy in corresponding to the ninth of Ab on the Hebrew calendar, a traditional Jewish fast day commemorating the destruction of the First and Second Temples in the Biblical era of Jerusalem.

National Institute of Allergy and Infectious Diseases, National Institutes of Health, Bethesda, MD 20892

Four months earlier, on March 31, in the grandeur of the former palace of the rulers of conquered Moorish Granada, the jointly reigning monarchs of Aragon and Castile, King Ferdinand and Queen Isabella, signed an edict expelling from their kingdoms all Jews who had not and would not convert to Catholicism. August 1 was fixed as the terminal date for completion of all matters pertaining to disposition of their properties, goods, and personal and business affairs, and for finalizing arrangements for their irreversible departure. Clearly in view was the lesson of horrors evoked by the ruthless and fervent pattern of the Spanish Church's Inquisition conducted in torture chambers and displayed in public festivals. Inhumane treatment and death, chiefly by burning at the stake, were visited upon scores of New Christians who were manipulated into confessing the sins of "Marranos" (Spanish, "swine"), those who secretly retained some Jewish religious practices. One hundred and fifty thousand Jews, from all walks of Spanish life and culture, chose to reject the proffered alternative of conversion.

On August 2, the last group forced to face the traumas and despair of expulsion and the rigors and hazards of travel in search of safe haven departed lifelong, generations-old homes and communities, and in many cases this was just the beginning of hardship and unscrupulous treatment. In ports of assembly and for passage on ships, they were often charged huge sums of money, sometimes several times over and for extra expenses that did not exist. Some shiploads of passengers were delivered to pirates in Africa and sold as slaves or offered for ransom to Jewish communities in Italy and France.

In stark contrast, August 2, 1492 was a gratifying day for Christopher Columbus to contemplate an optimistic future and the joy of a rewarding adventure ahead. Under the patronage of the Spanish sovereigns his ships were fully outfitted with crews in place and ready to embark. His projected expeditious approach to the wealth of the Orient was an undertaking far different in nature than the departing sea voyages for others beginning their forced exiles on that very day. On board in a harbor near Seville, shared with vessels taking on Jewish exiles, Columbus began his ship's log with an introductory entry (Fuson) addressing "Your Highness:"

> "as Catholic Christians and Princes devoted to the Holy Christian faith and to the spreading of it . . . (you) ordered that I should go to the east, but not by land as is customary. I was to go by way of the west, whence until today we do not know with certainty that anyone has gone."

particularly noting that:

> "Therefore, after having banished all the Jews from all your Kingdoms and realms, during this same month of January . . ."

If there was any sensitivity and appreciation of the plight of those who transiently entered into the record of Columbus' thoughts, it did not show as he continued.

> "Your Highnesses ordered me to go with a sufficient fleet to the said regions of India. For that purpose I was granted great favors and ennobled; from then henceforward I might entitle myself Don and be High Admiral of the Ocean Sea and Viceroy and perpetual Governor of all the islands and continental land that I might discover and acquire, as well as any other future discoveries in the Ocean Sea . . ."

Departure was deferred until the next day, and Columbus' fleet sailed out of Palos on August 3, 1492. Among the embarking Jews, whose exile Columbus noted, were some of Spain's leading physicians and scholars. Four years later an identical process of expulsion was duplicated in Portugal. With final banishment of the Spanish and Portuguese Jews, Europe's forefront of medicine and culture that had been nourished and advanced in the Iberian peninsula rapidly diminished.

There were many ironies apparent in these circumstances that embodied extremes of cruelty and favor, and suffering and indulgence. It was only through the direct involvements and assistance of descendants of Jewish blood lines that Columbus' voyage could be provided with the requisite means of support. The Spanish monarchs' unfavorable reception and rejection of Columbus' initial presentation had been reversed only because of the intervention of some forcibly converted Christians. The urging and proponent arguments initiated by Luis de Santagel and Gabriel Sanchez before Isabella gained substance in the huge sums offered by de Santagel, and another Aragon court-affiliated Jewish banker, Isaac Abravanel. The requisite support for Columbus's voyage materialized from their personal resources.

The critical nature of these contributions to the approval, support, and implementation of plans for the venture were underscored by Columbus' manner of recognition and appreciation, even though his written and subsequently published report of success was addressed to Santagel and Sanchez. Regardless of the important role Santagel had played in Ferdinand and Isabella's personal and State finances, religious zeal was more powerful. Members of Santagel's immediate family accused as Judaizers became victims of the Spanish Inquisition.

Insult was added to injury in the devious plan to add to the royal treasury by taking advantage of a spin-off benefit of the Inquisition's accomplishment. Penalties were levied on accused Marranos and whatever remained after they were put to death was confiscated. These seized assets furthered the Crown's venture of opening new lanes of commerce. With the finality of expulsion of the Jews completed on the eve of Columbus' embarkation, even more wealth that was left behind became available to stake on Spain's new agent en route to India and China. Jews were supposedly allowed to carry personal valuables with them, but this idea existed only in theory and was quite unattainable in practice, because the export of gold, silver and other precious metals was forbidden. Instant poverty for the fleeing translated into instant acquisition for Columbus' patrons to support his adventure.

Other Jewish-related contributions that enabled meeting needs of the fleet and its Admiral added to the irony of the voyage. Columbus' concept of sailing west to catch the trade winds to take his ship eastward derived from the astronomical tables developed by Abraham Zacuto, the famous Spanish-born, Portuguese Jewish physician, mathematician, and astronomer. The navigational instruments, upon whose use Columbus depended, were perfected by another Jewish physician-mathematician-astronomer, Joseph Vechino, who also was responsible for translating Zacuto's astronomic work into Spanish. The critical maps were produced through the special skills of the Jewish family of Mestre Jaime (Jafuda, Jehuda) Cresques, head of the school of cartography on the island of Majorca.

Some Marranos with the required sailing skills, whose motivation to join likely lay in the hope of finding escape from the Inquisition in China, have even been identified among Columbus' crew. There was Luis de Torres in the role of interpreter, for whom Columbus foresaw the need upon landing, even though de Torres' knowledge of languages was limited to Hebrew, Chaldean, and some Arabic. De Torres, a Jew hastily converted by baptism just before boarding, was the first of the Columbus expedition to set foot on American soil and to describe the natives' practice of smoking plant leaves and their cultivation of tobacco, which was subsequently introduced into Europe. Among the first Europeans to remain in the New World, De Torres settled in Cuba. Medical needs were served by the surgeon Marco and the ship's physician Mastro Bernal, both of Jewish stock. Just 2 years earlier, Bernal, as a Marrano adhering to Judaism, had been subjected by the Inquisition to a display of public penance.

Although Columbus would not live to see a further development, ultimately this simultaneously bright and dark period in history would take on an element of poetic justice. In time, Columbus' accidental encounter with newly found land would provide a meaningful response to the cloud over the spectacle of man's inhumanity to man under which the glorious voyage sailed. The exploring representatives of oppression had come upon a New World that would come to represent more than just territory. In yet another irony, the fruits of Ferdinand and Isabella's intolerance and persecution would offer the safety of new homes and opportunities for the victimized to rebuild shattered lives and careers for generations ahead. The continuation of contributions to medicine by Jewish physicians in distant lands was enhanced by the very societal forces that sought to destroy them.

GENESIS OF THE JEWISH PHYSICIAN

The image of practitioner of medicine is as old as the history of humane concerns and pursuits extending man's assistance to man in the Hebraic Old Testament. It quite naturally followed that the early emergence of Judaic physicians would place them in experienced positions of leadership, and often predominating and preeminent roles, in developing cultures.

Unlike the Egyptians who left behind medical papyruses, and the Greeks who recorded their medical opinions and dicta in special treatises, Hebrew scholars traditionally transmitted their funds of knowledge through the spoken word. The broad spectrum of religious historical lore provides informational insights into Biblical medicine, and compilations of the Palestinian and Babylonian Talmuds (sixth century B.C.–fifth century A.D.) paved the way for additionally revealing scholarly commentaries. By adopting monotheism as the unqualified principle of a structured religion, the Israelites were the first people to put aside the concepts of mysticism, magic, and superstition which formed

the empiric healing practices of their Egyptian, Assyrian, Babylonian, Greek, and Persian contemporaries. With Hebrew convictions that health and disease derived from a divine source and that man could only assume to serve as the conduit of God's will and command, religious beliefs and medical practices became intertwined. Public health came under the purview of priests, and agents of healing acted in roles of the spiritually endowed.

Employing objectivity, logic, disregard of mythology, and denial of a role for natural elements in the scheme of deities, religious leaders were involved in establishing hygienic codes and guidelines for preventive medicine. Within the Hebrew Bible are found accurate descriptions and identification of several diseases, the recognition of contagion and need for isolation, and references to items of materia medica and healing practices and regimes. Beyond its traditional base and hypotheses, Talmudic study of medicine employed critical observations, rational interpretations and analyses, and experimentation and autopsies on animals and humans.

In the Talmudic era, looking upon the physician's knowledge and skill as God's instruments of healing solidified the bridge between medicine and religion. The study of medicine was included in curricula and gave rise to Talmudic scholar-physicians and lines of rabbis whose pursuits combined both professions. An added benefit of this circumstance lay in ethical principles based upon teaching and study of the word of God—a pursuit of which should offer its own reward without consideration of monetary or other material gain. Such placement of responsibilities ensured giving the practice of medicine to the intellectually equipped, and provided an alternative acceptable means of support for rabbinical scholars.

In this setting Hebrew contributions were made to the new knowledge about anatomy, embryology, physiology, pathology, surgery, etiology, diagnosis, and therapy of disease. Against this background of development, advancement and recognition, Judaic physicians explored new vistas and experiences that would lead to Spain and Portugal.

ANTIQUITY: GREECE, ROME, AND BYZANTIUM

Coincident with the early and mid Talmudic periods, schools of thought and practice of healing based upon mythologic, magic, and astrologic concepts, and other ill-rationalized conjecture were taking shape in cultures outside Judea. In the Hellenistic world these conceptual offerings began with the appearance of a new breed of scholar who combined philosophy and the science of natural history as initiated by Thales (640–546 B.C.) and his pupil Anaximander (638–547 B.C). Pythagoras (580–489 B.C.) followed with the creation of a combined school of philosophy and religious cult in Sicily, then a Greek-Italian center of medicine founded by Empodocoles (493–433 B.C.). Subsequently mystic dogma gave way to the substantive collection of observations and precepts on health and disease as initiated by Hippocrates (460–370 B.C.) and the contributions of Aristotle (384–322 B.C.) to botany, zoology, and psychology.

An opportunity to solidify and centralize the recorded foundations of Greek science and medicine came with Alexander the Great's conquest of the Persian Empire and founding of the port city of Alexandria in 332 B.C. There, under Alexander's successor, Ptolemy, the development of a great library and museum began in 307 B.C. The Alexandria Library, in amassing a global collection of manuscripts and specimens, attracted large numbers of scholars focused on the teaching and study of science, technology, and medicine. Alexandria was preeminent as a center of intellectual creativity and training for physicians, engineers, geographers, astronomers, and mathematicians. For 200 years Alexandria enjoyed unique academic recognition, until the arrival of the Roman Legion under Julius Caesar in 48 B.C. sparked the first destructive strike.

With this eastward extension of Greek civilization to Egypt, just adjacent to Judea, cultural interactions and shared experiences in learning spread across geographic boundaries. Alexandrian tolerance and respect for the Israelites and their Hebrew religious traditions facilitated opportunities for Jews to resettle and engage in commerce and trade. Migrations from Palestine followed. With Judaic and Greek medicine introduced to each other, it is not surprising that Talmudic discussions make reference to a Judaic physician as a famous doctor from Alexandria (Bekhorot 4:4).

The opportunity thus arose for Jews to move westward, as well as eastward through earlier opened routes, beyond the Mediterranean site of fusion of Greek civilization and Egyptian lore in Alexandria. As Roman conquest and expansion followed Greek cultural influence, Palestinian emigrants during the first two centuries A.D. could be found established in Jewish communities in Rome and throughout the Roman Empire—Greece and the Greek islands, Italy, Spain, Gaul, Asia Minor, on the North African coast, on the shores of the Danube, and on the northern and southern coasts of the Black Sea. A number of factors led to Jewish expansion and settlements throughout the Arabian peninsula. These factors included an enlarging population that had outgrown the limited confines of Palestine, repeated invasions by Arab neighbors resulting in forced captivity and relocation, and defeat by Rome in 70 A.D. The Judaic scholar-physician thus came into practice throughout the then known civilized world.

In contrast to their experiences with Judaic medical and hygienic practices, Jewish settlers found the Roman search for health and healing set in a pattern of centuries-old precedents dependent upon temple objects, superstitious rites, and religious observances. Gradually, however, Roman medicine underwent transition as its practice was given to Greeks who were trained and experienced in the physician's craft.

The legacy of Hippocrates and the precepts set forth in the Hippocratic collection were gradually taken up, extended, and carried forward by successor Romans who gained fame as medical writers and physicians. Within the works of the historically renowned writer Aurelius Cornelius Celsus (25 B.C.–50 A.D.), the encyclopedist Gaius Plinius Secundis (Pliny the Elder) (23–79 A.D.), and the most prestigious and illustrious medical practitioner and investigator of all of Rome, Claudius Galen (130–200 A.D.), there are references to Jewish physicians and their skills and medicaments. The widespread reputations and high regard in which Jewish physicians were held are further exemplified by the eminence of those of other faiths whom they served, e.g., the Emperor Antonius Pius (86–161 A.D.), St. Basil (circa 300 A.D.), and Bishop Gelasius who was elevated to the papacy in 492 A.D. Nevertheless age-old discrimination was augmented as Christian bishops and emperors began to promulgate restrictions to which Jewish physicians were subject.

Because of Rome's priority on continuing militarism and conquest, and its diminishing concern for moral values, intellectualism and scientific search declined. With the loss of Greece, incentives for learning and teaching, and dedication to advancing philosophy and the arts began to suffer. Whatever remained of classic scholarship ultimately disappeared with the defeat and fall of the Western Roman Empire in the late fifth century. Progress in medicine could not escape inclusion among the casualties.

During the 250 years that followed Galen's death, there had not been a physician even resembling him in image or caliber, nor was there one of sufficient stature to replace his role, let alone extend or initiate innovative studies. Thus, centuries after Galen's lifetime and after Rome's waning years, the center of activity and importance drifted to the Eastern Roman Empire in Byzantium.

The teleologic tenor of Galen's concepts were held in high regard in Byzantium, and its culture displayed little interest in original search for specific facts. Emphasis was thus placed on Galen's Latin writings and they were translated into Greek as the language of Byzantine, and preserved and closely followed. Additionally, with large Persian and Syrian population segments, life in Byzantium was permeated by Eastern superstitions and mystic practices.

Since a major thrust of the Byzantine period (476–732 A.D.) was preservation of Greek culture, tradition and knowledge, both medicine and science remained static. Translations, rather than intellectual initiatives and generation of new knowledge, occupied the endeavors of dedicated physicians. A few of them additionally worked to compile the contributions of their Greco-Roman medical predecessors in systematic fashion. In these endeavors Jewish scholar-physicians played a major role. Although they lived under conditions of oppression, they worked with Jacobite and Nestorian Christian colleagues to save whatever was possible of Hellenistic heritage. Byzantine medical writers, e.g., Aetius of Amida (circa 550 A.D.) and Paulus of Aegina (625–690 A.D.) continued to refer to Jewish physicians.

The Persian invasion of Palestine in 611 A.D. and Mohammed's conquest of Mecca in 629 initiated the weakening of the Eastern Roman Empire. Its total disruption followed the Byzantine defeat at Yarmuk in 636 A.D. Within four years Islam took over Palestine and Syria. With their successful conquests, the Moslems found major Hebraic cultural contributions to medicine in place in their expanding domain.

Physicians who had evolved from rabbinical and Talmudic study in Judea and Babylonia had established their presence and skills throughout the mid East. One of the earliest to leave a mark in medical history was Asaf Judeus in sixth century Mesopotamia (modern day Iraq). In the oldest known medical textbook written in Hebrew, he produced an encyclopedic coverage of Greek, Babylonian, Persian, Egyptian, and Indian medicine with an incorporation of Hebraic medical techniques. Joined by colleagues, Asaf also founded a medical school. Other Jewish scholars, in the role of Byzantine translators, bridged centuries in the preservation of practical and theoretical aspects of medicine as described and pursued by preceding Greco-Roman multidisciplinary physician-philosophers. By transmitting accumulated knowledge, Jewish physicians and scholars were in position to play leading roles in the ascendancy of Arabic medicine.

THE ARABIC ERA

A rapid escalation of missionary zeal and military successes characterized the beginnings of the new religion introduced by the teachings of Mohammed (circa 570–632 A.D.). Out of the expansionist conquests of Mohammed's followers, Arab paganism was gradually replaced by an era of intellectual enlightenment. Jewish influences played a major contributory role in this cultural evolution and the ensuing progress in science and medicine.

Within a period of less than 100 years after Mohammed's cause got underway at Mecca and Yathrib (renamed Medina) in 622 A.D., Islam possessed virtually all of Arabia from Yemen to Syria, and Persia, Babylonia, Palestine, Egypt, and North Africa. Additionally it had spread to Asia at the northern border of

India, and across the Mediterranean to Spain and the south of France. While the physical forces of Jewish migration and Moslem invasion placed settlers of both peoples in the same lands, their subsequent interactions and joint pursuits took root in Hebraic-Islamic intellectual associations.

Because the essence of Mohammed's concepts and prophetic precepts, as set forth in the Koran, were based on Jewish principles of religion, morality, and ethics, Hebraic and Moslem beliefs and values had more similarities than disparities. Similarities included monotheism, shared Biblical origins traced to Abraham and Old Testament prophets, dietary codes, purity and cleanliness rituals, and rabbinical/mufti's responses or authority on points of law. Ultimately, however, magnification of minor differences came with a change in Mohammed's original design of Islam as an Arab version of Judaism. Combined with Moslem fervor aimed at forcing conversion of Jews, pagan Arabs, and Christians, attempts at subjugation won out. Once again Jews found themselves subjects of discrimination, and were required to pay heavy taxes, prohibited from building synagogues, riding horses, or carrying swords, and were forced to wear specified types of dress and identifying insignia. However, in most instances the pattern was not that of oppressive persecution as imposed under Christian domination, beause regulations were often relaxed or not strictly enforced. Most importantly under Moslem rule, Jews were permitted to maintain their own communities and live under their own religious governance. An ambience of tolerance generated mutual respect for intellectualism, utilization of knowledge, and exercise of skills.

The motivation and incentive for learning which the Moslems found in their contacts and interactions with eastern and western cultures of their new lands further enhanced the Jewish position. In viewing the philosophies passed along from ancient Greece and India, Islam came to appreciate the value, if not need, of attaining a literary and intellectual foundation. Through these avenues of stimulation, an Arabic cultural movement emerged to which the Jews had a natural attraction and capacity for contribution. Jewish poets wrote in Arabic and Jewish scholars translated Greek and Eastern language philosophic and scientific works into Arabic. Literate and industrious Jewish citizens rose to prominence as traders, bankers, and physicians. Some were welcomed into and selected for high level positions of trust and honor including those of personal and court physicians to ruling caliphs.

Medicine, intermixed with studies in ethics, philosophy, jurisprudence, natural science, mathematics, and the incentives for learning, flourished in the growing intellectualism of the new era. Known as the Arabic period of the Middle Ages, Arabist would be a more accurate characterization. The era was Arabic only insofar as the language in which the literature and cultural initiatives in this area largely were undertaken.

The revival of scientific medicine and responsibility for moving it forward began with the translators who worked to preserve Greek medical tradition. Here again Jewish physicians and scholars were at the forefront of advancement and spread of medical knowledge. They played important roles as primary teachers of Arabs in medicine and science until near the close of the ninth century when the Arabs themselves had advanced to the point of making noteworthy contributions. Centers were developed in the Jewish communities of El Faiyum in Egypt, Kairouan in Tunisia, and Cordova in Spain. At Arab hospitals and medical schools founded in Baghdad, Persia and Cairo, Jewish physicians joined in the work of Arab colleagues. In the absence of any Islamic laws prohibiting Jews to engage in medical practice, together with the Moslems they cultivated medicine.

Famous Jewish - Arabist Physicians

The recorded names of many Jewish physicians are noteworthy in the history of medicine's development during the Arabic period of the Middle Ages. Among some of the outstanding were the following. Masar Jawaih of Basra, who was physician to the Caliph Moawia and author of tracts on nutrition and medicinal plants in the first half of the seventh century. His translations from Syrian to Arabic were paramount in preserving early Moslem scientific writings. Ali-al Tabari Abu al-Hasan, a Persian Jew and Islamic convert, served as court physician to caliphs from 833 A.D. to 861 A.D. and wrote the first original Arabic medical textbook: *Paradise of Wisdom*. He gained fame as a renowned ophthalmologist and was the mentor of Rhazes (850–923 A.D.), who became the chief physician of the hospital at Baghdad and as a great clinician ranked alongside of Hippocrates and Aretaeus.

Isaac Judeus (Isaac ben Solomon Israel) (855–955 A.D.) was born in Egypt, studied in Baghdad, lived in North Africa, and excelled in logic, mathematics, astronomy, and medicine, and was especially authoritative and skilled in ophthalmology. His work influenced the great Persian physician Avicenna (980–1037 A.D.), who cited Isaac in his gigantic tome the *Canon of Medicine*. His writings on fever, diet, uroscopy, and ethics were the first Arabic works to be translated into Latin by the monk Constantinus Africanus (1020–1087 A.D.). They were the first Arabic-Latin translations to be introduced into Europe in Padua in 1487, and later were translated into Hebrew and Spanish. His books brought the influence of Hebraic-Arabic medicine to the countries of the Latin west and were regarded as classics for several centuries thereafter. Their influence continued with acceptance and use by the medical faculties in Vienna, Oxford, and Paris.

As a physician, philosopher, and rabbinical scholar, Maimonides (Moses ben Maimon) (1135–1204 A.D.) extended Hebrew learning beyond the Talmud and Talmudic commentaries by introducing science and philosophy into Jewish culture. He spent boyhood and early adult years in his native Cordova, but with the fading of Muslim tolerance his family fled Spain for Morocco. They later moved on to Palestine, and eventually Egypt. In Cairo, Maimonides entered the practice of medicine and rapidly rose to the position of Chief Physician to the court of the Sultan Salah Ed-Din Al-Ayyubi (Saladin). He wrote 10 treatises on a variety of medical subjects; the most famous included a *Treatise on Asthma*, two *Treatises on the Regimen of Health*, and the *Book of Precepts*.

In accordance with the state of the art of medieval medicine, Maimonides also subscribed to classical Greek teachings, but did not hesitate to depart from tradition. He criticized Galen when he found discrepancies and contradictions, warned against accepting blind beliefs, and emphasized the value of observation, experimentation, and logic in interpretation. Many of his commentaries were innovative and their validity stood the test of time.

The First Medical School

With the westward spread of Islam, the influence of Arabic medicine and the essence of its Greco-Roman foundation and tradition moved into southern Italy and Sicily. There an intermingling of the persisting Greek West and the more recently arrived Arab cultures furnished an arena for the entry of additional participants in intellectual pursuits. Contributions from immigrating Christian descendants of the earlier Hellenistic world of Syria and Egypt and members of the flourishing Italian Jewish communities added to the Greek, Latin, and Arabic ambience. In this milieu Europe's first medical school emerged in Salerno.

A small seaside town near Naples, Salerno had been well known as a health spa since the days of the Roman Empire. As an independent teaching and clinical center, it enjoyed cordial and cooperative relations with the Benedictine Hospital and monastery at nearby Monte Casino. There the School known as Civitas Hippocratica got underway during the ninth-tenth century. It later changed its name to the School of Salerno, and provided a setting of religious tolerance in which physicians and students flourished.

Since the founding of the School of Salerno, Jewish physicians were associated with its development. One named Joseph taught medicine at Salerno as early as 848 A.D. and another named Joshua taught in 885 A.D. Physician and astrologer Sabbato Dunnolo (913–982) of Orio, Calabria, the first European Jew to write a Hebrew language medical treatise, is mentioned in conjunction with the founding of the school. His text on pharmacology, *The Precious Book*, contained remedies consisting of drugs and spices Jews had brought from the East. There are records of the use of Hebrew as a language of instruction, and references to Jewish physicians and teachers continuing in Salerno into the 11th–12th centuries, when the school had enough graduates to replenish its faculty. In nearby Naples under Frederick II (1194–1250) lectures in medicine were also given in Hebrew.

Salerno's vitality preserved the basis and tradition of medical practice launched during the classical centuries. Its cultural effect stood in contrast to the intellectual stagnation, dearth of medical knowledge, and primitive, mystic, and fraudulent practices that characterized Europe in the Dark Ages. By the time of the School of Salerno's beginning decline in the early 13th century, Salerno and the westward movement of Hebrew-Arabic culture and medicine had influenced the development of medicine in universities and medical centers in the Italian cities of Bologna, Padua, and Naples, and in Sicily and Montpelier in southern France.

During the Middle Ages, Jewish physicians found acceptance in Christian Europe only as long as they were found useful. From the time Zedekius (d. 880 A.D.), the first registered Jewish physician in Franco-Germany, served Louis the Pious (814–840 A.D.) and his son Charles the Bald (843–877 A.D.), Jewish physicians flourished beyond the Arabic sphere. As Hebrew-Latin translators, they brought the Arabic and Greek medical literature to Europe. As teachers and practitioners they were at the forefront in providing care and introducing new ideas.

Based on a background of considerable experience in the treatment of eye diseases, which were prevalent in nearby Eastern countries, Jewish physicians filled the void of oculists that had existed in European countries. Even the pioneering medieval university faculties of medicine in Bologna, Padua, and Paris could not provide instruction in ophthalmology at that time. Introduction of the teaching of ophthamology as a separate discipline in European university clinics came in the early 19th century in Germany at Göttingen. There were two important factors that led to the Jewish and Moslem physicians gaining the requisite skills and expertise. First was the high prevalence of varied types of eye diseases in the mid-East with which medical practitioners were faced. Second was the development of mathematics in the Arabic era and sphere and the insights for applying mathematical principles to optical phenomena.

Usually regarded as having superior scientific knowledge, the Jewish and Moslem physicians practiced under the personal protection of kings, popes, and nobles. Their successes and attainments were largely derived from therapeutic practices based on established fact and knowledge, and stood in contrast to the approach of Christian counterparts who were influenced by superstition. However, when these physicians were no longer needed in particular roles, appreciation gave way to bigotry. Exemplifying this circumstance was the action of the Council of Vienna, which in 1267 forbade the practice of Jewish physicians among Christians, and the closing of Montpelier to Jews in 1301.

Only in the Islamic held territories of the East, Arabia, North Africa, and Moorish Spain did Moslem and Jew live in mutually supportive and tolerant circumstances of common respect for culture and knowledge. In addition to serving the Islamic communities, schools, and hospitals, Jewish physicians were appreciated in roles of personal and court services to caliphs and emirs. Nevertheless, life for the Jew was not without periodically recurring problems. Their rejection of Mohammed as the true prophet neither could be understood nor forgiven by Moslem neighbors and hosts. One consideration, however, remained overriding—the rewarding Jewish contribution to the harmony, development, and progress of Hebraic-Arabic medicine and the shared images of Jewish and Arab physician-philosopher-scientist. This consideration would pass all too soon. Christian Spain, the Catholic Kings Ferdinand and Isabella, and 1492 lay ahead.

SPAIN IN TRANSITION FROM MOSLEM TO CHRISTIAN

The Moslem bridging of the Mediterranean from North Africa to the west and the expansion of Islam's domain to Spain in 744 A.D. provided seeds for growth of a period of heightened culture in the newly conquered land. It was a period of splendor and achievement known commonly as the "Golden Age." With its beginnings the door was opened for extending the Arabic-Hebraic pattern of life. With it came new opportunities for Jewish economic, religious, and scholarly pursuits in Spain, a land where these avenues had previously been barred.

Under the Visigoth kings, who had taken up Roman Catholicism, the rule was persecution. Jews were flogged, executed, oppressively taxed, forcefully baptized, forbidden to follow their religion, and barred from engaging in trade. Eleven years before the Moslem invasion, by decree anyone found practicing a Jewish ceremony was sold into slavery and his or her children turned over to the Church to be raised by the clergy. Those who elected to accept conversion as the only possible escape, but who became Christian in name only, introduced the secret Jew, the Marrano, into Spanish life and history. A far greater number, almost the entire Jewish population, was driven out. With their exodus, whatever of Biblical, Talmudic Hebraic, and Greek medicine the Jewish physician had brought with the earlier Roman Empire's penetration and establishment of western provinces, disappeared from Spain.

A transplanted Jewish community that had taken refuge in North Africa, waiting to return from exile, saw the opportunity to return materialize in 711 A.D. with the Moslem invasion of Spain. Jewish alliances assisted both the advancing armies of Islam and the planting of Arabic culture in the overrun lands. As Jews established themselves in conquered Spanish cities, they found the same ambience of tolerance and benevolence they had enjoyed under the caliphs of Baghdad, Kairowan in Tunisia, and Fez in Morocco. In Cordoba, Granada, Toledo, and Seville there were opportunities for economic advancement as traders, craftsmen, and bankers and for scholarly pursuits as physicians. Open routes to a gracious and productive way of life attracted immigration from Persia and Babylonia.

The influence of Arabic-Hebraic shared respect and appreciation for cultural objectives was exemplified by Caliph Abd al-Rahman III (897–961 A.D.) of the Ummayid dynasty and his Jewish court physician-astronomer-diplomatic advisor Hisdai ibn Shaprut (915–970 A.D.). Hisdai's considerable stature was further enhanced by his gratefully received contribution of a translation from Latin to Arabic of Dioscorides' widely accepted work on materia medica. Through Hisdai's influence, Jewish scholars, philosophers, scientists, and poets were brought to Cordoba to make it a leading cultural center. Toledo also gained fame as the center for translators of Arabic science and literature into Latin, Hebrew, and Castilian. Through Semitic intellectual resources and activity, the essences of ancient and Arabic culture and Greek and Arabic medicine were preserved and transmitted to Christian Europe. Toledo produced Judah-ha-Levi (circa 1086), remembered as one of history's greatest Hebrew poets, whose work in several languages is still available and read.

Spain, especially in its Jewish communities, was propelled into a golden period of freedom, wealth, splendor, and achievement. Literature, art, science, and philosophy were encouraged and flourished. Schools, libraries, and scientific societies were founded, and industrial and agricultural developments undertaken. Jews and Moors in joint participation cultivated medicine and built hospitals. Characteristic of the age was the combination of multidisciplinary secular and religious scholarship. Thus among a lengthy list of Spain's historically prominent there were those who were simultaneously rabbis and physicians and practiced at high societal levels. Like their scholarly Arabic contemporaries, they distinguished themselves as philosophers, mathematicians, astronomers, translators, poets, grammarians, and authors. In the courts of kings, emirs, and caliphs, some Jewish physicians even served beyond these roles as advisors and viziers. Unfortunately, after three glorious centuries of intellectual freedom and contributions to educational and cultural advancement, destructive diminishing forces again took over.

The 300 years of favorable rapport and partnership for Arabic-Jewish world of enlightenment began to wane in the 10th century. Within the Mohammedan principalities that formed in North Africa and Spain independent of earlier central governance in Baghdad, escalating conceptual and philosophic differences reached the breaking point. A series of invasions and takeovers by North African tribes bought a new brand of fanatic Islamic fundamentalism to Spain. First it was the Ahmoravides, who began their rule in 1086 A.D. and created difficulties by insisting on conversion. When they were replaced by the conquering Almohads in 1148, Islamic zeal and punishment of nonbelievers who would not accede to forced conversion was pushed even further to an extreme. Synagogues and schools were demolished and Jewish wives and children were sold into slavery. Once again the Jews attempted to escape persecution by fleeing, this time heading north to the Christian area of Spain and westward to France.

It was during this period that Maimonides, who otherwise might have given his talents and abilities to Spanish medicine, left Cordoba to rise to fame as court physician to the Sultan Saladin in Cairo. Scholars who escaped to the southeastern region of France known as Provence made historically noteworthy contributions to French intellectualism and literary activity and to development of the University of Montpelier in 1181 A.D. Jewish physicians trained in the Moorish schools of Spain played major roles as teachers in the founding of Montpelier's facility of medicine. One of their number, Jacob ben Mahir, became Dean in 1300 of what today is recognized as the world's oldest existing medical school.

The second factor in the Arabic-Jewish cultural dissolution was the progressive growth of the early small Christian enclaves that the Moslem invaders originally allowed to remain in the northern mountainous regions of Spain. Gaining increasing strength and forging contacts with France, the independent kingdoms of Castile, Aragon, Navarre, Leon, and Portugal emerged. By the end of the 11th century they had achieved their own identities and began to expand their territorial holdings by moving militarily against the Moors. With the added advantage of the internal strife that divided the Moslem factions, in 1212 the Spanish kingdoms defeated the Almohads in battle, and by 1248 took over Islam's Spanish dominion. Only the small southernmost Moorish kingdom of Granada remained where Jews could continue living in Spain unmolested in their work and study. In Granada they continued to enjoy cultural pursuits, practice medicine, and serve as physicians to the king. In 1492 that chapter too would come to a tragic end.

In the early developmental years of the Spanish Christian kingdoms, the Jews found their lot quite comfortable while practical applications of their special knowledge and pursuits were useful to the kings. In most instances their capabilities, financial holdings, taxable wealth, and experiences as traders, merchants, and bankers, and their intellectual attainments as scholars and court advisors loomed paramount. They became almost indispensable. The kings depended upon Jewish subjects for income and the type of political support that was not given by Christian antagonists who constituted the ambitious and self-serving provincial nobility. The loyalty and dependability of Jewish subjects earned them appointments as treasurers and tax collectors.

Further realizing the special advantages inherent in professions that offered mobility, status, and dependence of others upon their skills, the most able Spanish Jews were attracted to the practice of medicine. Virtually every Christian monarch appointed one or more highly regarded Jewish physicians as his personal doctor. The confidence placed in them and the superiority and advantages they enjoyed over Christian counterparts were justly earned. Basic programs of solid instruction in several languages and sciences in the Jewish schools of Spain were enhanced by opportunities to develop self-discipline and moral values. The endeavors of Jewish physicians were unlike Christian professional contemporaries. They were unique in gaining indepth knowledge of the medical treatises of antiquity, in developing a proper system of therapeutics, and in sorting out factual and established principles of medical practice from superstitious and mystical concepts. In keeping with the culture of the times some Jewish physicians, through appointments by their patron kings, also served concurrent roles as chief rabbis of their religious constituencies, political counselors, and in scholarly posts such as official astronomers and mathematicians. They enjoyed the protection and support of reigning Christian monarchs even if for no reason other than to serve the king's self-interest.

Thus, the ascendancy of Jewish-Spanish culture that began three centuries earlier in the Hebraic-Islamic alliance was carried into Catholic Spain. The great promise and potential in Spain continued during the early Moslem to Christian transitional years. In 1243 the university in Salamanca, and 4 years later the one in Seville, joined the list of European medieval universities that began with the foundings of the first faculties in France (Paris 1110), Italy (Bologna 1113), and England (Oxford 1167), but the "Golden Age" was not to last. Preoccupation with the demands of the war years had diverted the Spanish Christian population from intellectual priorities for too long. With little in the way of stimulation and incentive compounded by church-oriented bias, the cultural level that otherwise could have been the Moslem-Hebrew legacy, declined. In this setting the same admirable societal, economic, and professional attainments that engendered royal protec-

tion, confidence, and trust for Jewish subjects, in time provided cause for their erosion.

There were quite evident similarities in the patterns of relationships for Jewish life under Moslem caliphs and Christian kings. Challenges to religious and personal freedom and threats to life did not originate within the royal purviews, but rather at peer and lower levels. Although Jews had lived in Spain and contributed to its growth and development as long as had their Christian neighbors, as a minority they were considered "outsiders." Christian artisans and merchants disdained their Jewish counterparts as successful competitors, and the nobility envied their acquisition of wealth. As creditors and recipients of favors and in positions of prominence granted to nonbelievers, they were resented by all. In no circumstance was this more demonstrable than among physicians. The fact that Jewish physicians were widely popular, were called upon with frequency, served in high positions, and were considered especially skillful, motivated attacks by Christian colleagues. Attempts at elimination were made through the encouraging adoption of practice restrictions and professional defamation. In hostility and anti-Jewish actions Christian medieval colleagues rivaled Catholic monks.

The Christian kings often took strong positions in favor of their Jewish subjects at court levels, even to the extent of opposing papal edicts. As long as the Jews had economic strength and resources to contribute, they were excused from wearing church-imposed brands e.g., yellow patches displayed on outer garments. Ultimately, however, levels of Christian endeavors caught up in trades, administration, and intellectual accomplishments. By the 13th century the kings, in order to minimize threats of impending rebellion, could now afford to look the other way. Open instances of bodily attacks, riots, destruction of property, legal injustices, ignoring debts and contracts, and other dishonest financial practices occurred unopposed with frequency.

As a consequence there were increasing conversions to Catholicism, both forced and voluntary. However distasteful, conversion became accepted as the last and only means of escaping severe oppression and/or of preserving life, property, and centuries of heritage. The Jewish population steadily decreased. Whatever remained of the Jewish potential for scientific, societal, and educational contributions passed into the hands of the Marranos. With dissipation of the country's earlier attained level of culture, there was little left in the way of intellectual stimulation or opportunities to engage Spain's Jewish communities. The "Golden Age" fell into rapid decline.

Nevertheless Jewish physicians continued to hold a very special place in Spanish civil life. No matter that the Church threatened danger to the soul of a patient who called upon a Jewish physician. Such ethereal risks did not prevent Christians from seeking the practical help of a Jewish medical expert when faced with the more earthly danger of illness. Jewish physicians, whenever available, continued to be called upon preferentially by Christian patients, especially by those among high ranking members of both the nobility and clergy.

Until the Inquisition and the Edict of Expulsion tragically finalized the fate of Spanish Jews, there were diametrically opposite forces at play— benevolence versus persecution, and monarchy versus church. As a result a complexity of paradoxes and mixed messages presented an ever-changing picture. An early representation of this development was seen in Pope Gregory VII's epistle in 1080 admonishing Alfonso VI of Castile (1073–1109) for his display of friendliness and utilization of Jewish talents as court physicians, viziers, chancellors, and army officers. This in Gregory's view was subordinating Christians to Jews, equivalent to oppressing God's church and exalting Satan's synagogue. Papal pronouncements led to repressive laws. The first was framed between 1256–1265 and forbade Christians to take medicines or purges from Jews unless prescribed by a learned Jew and prepared by a Christian who understood the substances. At provincial levels, a series of 14th century Church councils struck out for control. From Zamora in 1313, Jewish physicians were not to practice among Christians. From Salamanca in 1322, Christians were not to employ Jewish physicians, surgeons, or apothecaries or take their medicines; and from Valladolid in 1322, Christians were forbidden to accept medical aid from Jews and Saracens.

Repetitiously the synods (e.g., Beziers in 1255, Vienna in 1267, Avignon in 1326, Bamberg in 1491) issued warnings that it was preferable for Christians to die rather than to owe their lives to Jews. These periodic identical admonitions were likely provoked by the continuing priority that those in positions of authority gave to retaining their appointed Jewish physicians over Church edicts that posed threats to their personal welfare. Just as Jewish physicians accepted conversions, even if only for the sake of survival, many Spanish and Portuguese patrons also went through the motions of paying lip service to decrees. Jew and Gentile shared a show of pretense and deception to support each others' needs.

The complexity and paradoxical nature of a spectrum of varied relationships and attitudes are exemplified in the saga of the Spanish and Portugese kings and their Jewish physicians that follow (Kagan; Friedenwald).

Castile

Putting aside Church attempts to influence or control self-serving interests, a long line of Castilian kings continued to give substance to their beliefs in the unique skills, talents, intellects, and traditions the Jews had brought to medical practice. Not only were Jewish physicians prominent in personal and court roles, the thread of sensitivity and appreciation running through successive reigns was evident in the special privileges and exemptions granted to them.

Although he initially curtailed Jewish rights and liberties, Alfonso VII (1126–1157) subsequently came under the influence of his Jewish physician and household majordomo, Judah ben Joseph ibn Ezra. In a reversal of earlier hostility, Alfonso's subsequent actions granted equality to his Jewish and Christian subjects. Also among the early benevolent was Alfonso VIII (1158–1214), despite the letter of reproof he received from Pope Innocent III for showing tolerance to his Jewish subjects.

In a paradoxical circumstance Alfonso X The Wise (1252–1284) incorporated into his codes of law the Church's most intolerant laws, yet at the same time he was reproached by Pope Nicholas III for showing preference to Jews. Curiously, while Alfonso X had a Jewish personal physician, Judah ben Moses ha-Kohen, he fostered the legal principle that Christians should not take medications prepared by a Jew. In a noteworthy contribution to Spanish science and medicine, Alfonso X provided the requisite patronage to Jewish physicians and translators to prepare and publish the entire body of Arabic knowledge in Castilian Spanish. Both Alfonso and his son Ferdinand III (1217–1252) conferred the title of Nasi (Prince) upon their respective personal physicians, also father and son, Joseph and Judah Al-Fakar.

When the position of the Castilian Jews became especially endangered following the edicts of the Zamora, Salamancan, and Valladolid Councils, Alfonso XI (1312–1350), whose court favorite was a Jewish physician, did much to restore a measure of reason and tranquility. His son Pedro I (1350–1369) followed in the same pattern of Jewish associations and favorable treatment to the extent that opponents ridiculed him for his "Jewish Court." In 1367 the Cortes (Assembly) presented Pedro with a petition to bar any Jew from the position of physician, officer, or any post in the household of the King, Queen, or their families. Purported reasons were the evils, misfortunes, murders, and banishments blamed on influential Jewish advisors who through successive reigns had wished to harm and injure Christians. Although Pedro refused to yield to these demands and continued to retain Jews in palace positions, he did propose to keep them out of councils and away from positions of power where they might do damage. Even more contradictory was the behavior of Henry II (1369–1379) whose antagonism to his half-brother Pedro I was extended to those whom Pedro appreciated and protected. In the process of overthrowing Pedro, Henry subjected Jews to robbery, butchery, and murder. Nevertheless during his reign, Henry bent to self-serving interests and kept Jews on as physicians, tax collectors, and financial counselors.

Henry III's succession in 1390 was characterized by a complete breakdown of law, order, and justice. Murderous riots erupted and a number of clerical Jew-baiters arose to lead the agitation. The Dominican Vincente Ferrer (1350–1419) led a typical mission of breaking into synagogues and dedicating them as churches. There is no record of any Jews in Henry's court and restrictions were cast into law.

The terror that was generated during the reign of Henry III (1390–1406) was compounded by his son Juan II (1406–1454). In 1411 a proclamation let it be known that the king ordered and judged it right that Jews and Moors should not be physicians, surgeons, apothecaries, accoucheurs, or nurses—whether to the great or the small. In addition to barring Jews from medical and surgical practice, Juan imposed severe restrictions on both Jewish and converso (converted) tradesmen alike, especially dealers in herbs and food stuffs. Christians had to be protected against the poisons that these traders and dealers could and would supposedly spread through their products. Ironically, at the same time Juan and members of his court favored Jewish physicians. Juan's position in this hypocritical circumstance is seen in a statement to the effect that neither canon nor state law forbid Christians from taking medical advice from Moorish or Jewish physicians provided Christians prepared the medications.

In some of the most hostile and depriving acts, special exceptions and privileges were afforded to physicians. Juan I (1371–1390) was responsible for a Council decree that no Christian might associate with, entrust with office, or have in his home any Jew or Moor, except a physician when required. This was a convenient edict for Juan to follow since his own longstanding trusted physician, Moses ibn Zarzal, was Jewish. In 1481 in Madrid, an exception to live outside the ghetto was granted to the Jewish city physician so that he could be called at night when the ghetto was locked. In 1482, the Tafalla Cortes ordered Jews to remain at home and off the streets on Sundays and holidays, except physicians and surgeons so that they could visit their patients.

Even Isabella and Ferdinand, who were responsible for the nadir of Spanish humanity through the Inquisition and Act of Expulsion, were at the forefront of hypocrisy. Isabella herself had a Jewish physician to whom she granted special privileges and tax exemption in appreciation of his services. In 1490, Ferdinand (Fernando) granted permission to a Jewish physician to be examined for approval to practice, and revealed the two sides of his belief. He noted that although it was necessary to refute and repulse Jewish nonbelievers, it would be absurd not to accept them where, without injuring one's faith or health of soul, they could aid in the condition of a Christian's body.

In the dichotomies of prejudice versus special consideration and persecution versus special privilege, the leadership of the Church was similarly represented. Despite Council edicts and Papal bulls proclaiming that Christians should not use the services of Jewish physicians or the medications of Jewish apothecaries or compounders of drugs, the practice of ecclesiastical medicine continued to be predominantly in Jewish hands until the time of the Spanish expulsion. Even higher clergy were too concerned for their own needs to give more than lip service to canonically-imposed restrictions.

During periods of this era that varied in contrasting degrees of papal benevolence and hostility, there were bishops whose personal physicians were Italian Jews. Among these prominent bishops were Popes Nicholas IV (1287–1292) and Boniface IX (1392). As late as 1460, a Franciscan friar and leading Jew-baiter Alfonso de Spina accompanied his comment on the Christians' neglect of the study of the art of medicine with a lament. He noted that ecclesiastic prelates put such store in Jewish practitioners that there was hardly one of rank that did not harbor a "devil of a Jewish doctor" and in turn serve as advocate and defender for the accused.

In the mid 14th century the epidemic plague that swept across Europe added fuel to provoked attacks. Anti-semitic clergy stirred up crowd anger and pointed to the Jews as agents of the Black Death, who in alliance with the Devil, poisoned the wells. In an attempt to stop the ensuing massacres of Jews, Pope Clement VI issued a bull declaring the Jews innocent of charges and rationally pointed to the fact that they shared equally in the suffering and ravages of the disease. Among other outrageous inflammatory charges made against Jewish physicians was the accusation that they sacrificed Christian children to recover their blood for use in religious, symbolic, and ceremonial foods.

In 1388 when Archbishop of Toledo and Primate of Spain, Di Pedro Tenario designated his physician Hayyim ha-levi to be Chief Rabbi and Judge of the Toledo congregations, the King upheld and confirmed the appointment. In contrast to the harsh restrictions imposed by Juan I (1371–1390) including the prohibition of any physician or surgeon among the Jews, excepting the King's physician, Pope Martin I in 1421 issued a bull granting Jewish physicians permission to practice in Spain.

During the reign of Henry IV (1454–1474) conditions for the Jews of Castile were returned to a more favorable state. Although Henry confirmed an earlier law that prohibited Jews from positions as apothecaries or compounding drugs for Christians, he employed several Jewish physicians whom he exempted from taxation. The relatively tranquil and comfortable 20-year period under Henry came to an end when Isabella succeeded her half-brother in 1474.

Aragon

Similar to the trend and tradition so visible in the courts of neighboring Castile, the Christian kings of Aragon employed Jewish personal physicians. However, quite in contrast to Castile, Aragon's political climate made it easier to sustain the personal privileges and tolerance Jewish scholars and other contributing members of the community enjoyed for several centuries. From its beginning identity as an evolving Spanish kingdom in the 11th–12th centuries, Aragon was more liberal than Castile.

The earliest kings of Aragon, Alfonso II and Pedro II, gave special grants during the late 12th–early 13th centuries to their Jewish physicians. James I (1213–1276) had several Jewish physicians and surgeons, and even succeeded in gaining the agreement of Pope Honorius III to bestow special favors and honors on them. To one of them, Isaac of Barcelona, Honorius in 1220 additionally extended the shelter of papal protection. To another, Benveniste, he sent a diploma conferring "Catholicorum Studiosus" with exemption from all indignities; henceforth the family name of Benveniste would appear with frequency among Spain's leading physicians. During a subsequent papal tenure, Clement IV in 1265–1266 demanded the removal of the many Jewish officials whom James had engaged, but the King would not yield. James further defied and angered the Pope by repudiating his first wife and bodily attacking the papal representative, the Bishop of Gerona. James' open-mindedness and fairness was especially demonstrated by the manner in which he set up and conducted public debate. Whereas the formal disputations, which were introduced in France in 1240 and continued in Spain and other European countries during the Middle Ages, were designed as staged baiting confrontations, James did not subscribe to this arrangement. In 1263 in Barcelona he set the model for genuine Christian-Jewish discussion on valid points of doctrine with the guarantee of free speech. Furthermore, he recruited and honored a famous learned rabbi and physician Moses ben Nachman (Nachmanides) to speak for the Jewish position.

That the entrusting of health to the care of Jews extended beyond the Crown was seen in the writing of Raymond Lully (1235–1315), who was both famous as a distinguished physician of his time and a violent antisemite. Noting that almost every monastery had its Jewish physician, he called attention to the guilt of the Church in such an abomination and accursed custom.

Special privileges and favored treatment, along with preferences for and employment of Jewish physicians, were displayed through several successive reigns—from Pedro III (1276–1285) to Juan II (1458–1479). Examples included exemption from taxes, legal pardons, exemption from wearing identifying Jewish cloaks and badges, admission to examinations, and authorization to practice medicine. In 1397 when King Martin's (1395–1410) wife Queen Maria issued a decree in his absence forbidding Jewish physicians to treat Christian patients, the King countermanded the action on his return to the country.

A diverting influence from this trend of rational coexistence appeared when the bigoted voice of the Dominican monk Vincent Ferrer (circa 1350–1419) found a receptive audience. Exceeding the effect of his drive to break into synagogues and force conversion of the congregants under threat, Ferrer and his clerical colleagues sought to make the Church and State official allies. The objective was achieved by engineering the selection of a new king, Ferdinand I, in 1412, to implement their contrived anti-Jewish policies and gain the approval of Pope Benedict XIII.

In the next king, Alfonso V (1416–1458), however, rival Jewish interests once again found a champion. Among the rights Alfonso granted to Jews were acceptance as physicians and surgeons and the treatment of Christians. As a result of just consideration and gracious protection under the Crown, Jewish physicians and surgeons flourished in Aragon as practitioners, writers, translators, and contributors to medical and scientific information.

This last, although a declining vestige of the Golden Age, would end with the conclusion of the reign of Juan II (1458–1479). Juan expressed great gratitude to a Jewish ophthalmologist Abiatar Cresques who had successfully operated on his bilateral cataracts and restored his vision. When Juan was succeeded by Fernando II (Ferdinand), physicians shared in the repressions, suffering, and death that the age of the Inquisition and expulsion visited upon Spain's Jewish community.

Navarre

With the separation of Portugal from Spain in 1112 and the union of Leon with Castile in 1230, Navarre was the only remaining independent Iberian Christian kingdom until it was occupied by Castile in the the early 16th century. Beginning in 905 A.D. with the first king, Sancho I, through Sancho VII the Wise and Sancho VIII the Strong (1194–1234), Navarre's Jews enjoyed royal protection and consideration. Jewish physicians were given court positions and rewarded. A hiatus from favored status then followed during a period of French domination (1284–1328).

In the mid 14th century references to Jewish physicians again appeared, especially in relationship to valued services rendered to Carlos III (1387–1425). His expressions of appreciation included gifts of houses and annual payments and pensions. The confidence Jewish physicians enjoyed was exemplified by Carlos' physician and Grand Rabbi of Navarre, Juze Orabuena, who accompanied the King on trips and prolonged visits in France. Similarly a few years later Juan I had his physician Maestre Jacob Abocar accompany him on a pilgrimage.

Although it could afford some protection, the position of king's physician could often place the Jewish holder in jeopardy. The physicians were required to take oaths to faithfully perform medical duties, guard the king's person, hinder and give notice of any attempted injury to him, and keep entrusted information sacred. Despite the favorable tone set by the kings, Jews were subjected to escalating acts of degradation, brutality, and persecution by unenlightened masses. Nevertheless the presence of a good number of Jewish physicians, scholars, and philosophers gave testimony to sustaining intellectual freedom. In 1392 a decree of the Cortes restricted Jews to their quarters on Sundays, holidays, and during hours of Church services. Physicians and surgeons, however, were exempted so that patients could be attended. This provision underscored both the importance of the Jewish physician and the dichotomy of considerations when Spanish individual self-interests needed to be served. By 1492 Navarre's decline became more obvious and ultimately finalized when occupied by Castile in 1512.

BIBLIOGRAPHY

Dale PM. Christopher Columbus. In: The Ailments of Thirty-three Famous Persons. Norman, OK: University of Oklahoma Press, 1952, pp. 16–19.

Encyclopedia Judaica. Volume II, Medicine. Jerusalem: Keter Publishing House, 1971, pp. 1178–1196.

Friedenwald H. The Jews and Medicine, Essays. Baltimore: Johns Hopkins Press, 1944.

Fuson RH. The Log of Christopher Columbus (English translation). Camden, ME: International Marine Publishing Company, 1987.

Grangel LS, Palermo JR. Medicina y sociedad en la espana renacentista. In: Historia Universal de la Medicina. Entralgo PL, ed. Barcelona: Salvat Editores, 1973, pp. 181–189.

Grayzel S. A History of the Jews. Philadelphia: Jewish Publication Society, 1968.

Johnson P. A History of the Jews. New York: Harper and Row, 1987.

Kagan SR. Jewish Contributions to Medicine in America. Boston: Boston Medical Publishing Company, 1939.

Kagan SR. Jewish Medicine. Boston: Medico-Historical Press, 1952.

Kayserling M. Christopher Columbus and the Participation of Jews in the Spanish and Portugese Discoveries. Translated by Gross C, 4th ed. New York: Hermon Press, 1968.

Kayserling M. Sephardim, Romanische Possien der Juden in Spanien. Leipzig: 1859.

Perry ME, Cruz AJ, eds. Cultural Encounters, The Impact of the Inquisition in Spain and the New World, Berkeley: Univ Calif Press, 1991.

Rise GR. Medicine in New Spain. In: Medicine in the New World. Numbers RL, ed. Knoxville: University of Tennessee Press, 1987, pp. 12–63.

Sokoloff L. Rise and decline of Jewish quota in medical school admissions. Bull NY Acad Med, in press.

Wiesenthal S. Sails of Hope: The Secret Mission of Christopher Columbus. Translated by Winston C, Winston R. New York: Macmillian, 1973.

Yerushalmi YH. From Spanish Court to Italian Ghetto. Isaac Cardoso: A Study in Seventeenth Century Marranism and Jewish Apologetics. New York: Columbia University Press, 1971. □

Spain, Portugal, Christopher Columbus, and the Jewish Physician: The Inquisition and Expulsion

Sheldon G. Cohen, M.D.

THE INQUISITION AND EXPULSION

"Men never do evil so completely and cheerfully as when they do it from religious conviction."

Blaise Pascal, *Pensées*, No. 894 (1670)

A force that had begun as discrimination based on envy and resentment of the wealth, success, and position attained by industrious, intellectual, and cultured Jews gained momentum with the zealous encouragement of early 14th century Church Council decrees. Anti-Jewish agitators escalated bigotry into acts of persecution, and in 1391 incited mobs to riots and massacres in Seville, Cordoba, and Toledo. As violence and mass killings spread to Catalonia, Barcelona, Majorica, and Aragon, the groundwork was laid for the Inquisition and destruction of Spanish Jewry. Whether economically, socially, or religiously inspired, overt zeal for anti-Semitism was taken up by all classes, at all levels, and in all walks of life.

Into the 15th century there were few enclaves of safety, sensitivity, and understanding for Jewish physicians beyond the royal courts they attended. Logically, with the augmented trust, confidence, dependence, and appreciation represented by the level of the position given by a king or royal dignitary, one would expect augmented protection for the Jewish physician by his patron; however, this parallel degree of security did not invariably follow.

The price to be paid for achievment was increased visibility and enhancement of the hated Jewish image. Targeted hostility was directed even beyond individuals to their colleagues and the communities with which they were identified. Jewish physicians offered a personal service to royalty. The taxable Jewish community and the resources of Jewish financiers offered a broader base of economic value. Nevertheless, sometimes these priority interests had to be sacrificed for purposes of appeasement. There was always the possibility that disgruntled middle-class anti-Semitic townspeople might turn to independent nobles whose motivation for opposition was always a threat to the king and thus not be trusted. For the sake of temporary expediency, attacks on Jews could be overlooked, repressive rules issued, and accusations answered by approving executions and confiscating properties. Depending on factors of locale, position, circumstance, and governance the rights and privileges of medical practice were subject to variable and cyclic fluctuations.

While riots and attacks succeeded in destroying Jewish lives and property, they did not accomplish the objective of diminishing Judaism. Many Jews were so devoted to their faith that they preferred death to conversion. Others, especially those belonging to the upper class, elected to take their chances as Christians and adapt to Catholicism's requirements. Many hoped to revert or escape when opportunities arose or to secretly retain Jewish religious practices. Following the dictates of conversion and fitting into the new mode of religious life did not come either automatically or easily. The Church not only had other ideas; it created an insoluble problem. In all out efforts to convert the Jews, it depicted them as having such dark genetic traits of character that once converted their fellow Christians found it impossible to understand how they could be trusted. Any deviation from absolute devoutness and sincerity could not be tolerated; questionable New Christians would have to be rooted out and punished. Within the religious community, to whose demands the converted now were required to profess unqualified loyalty and belief, there invariably were fellow Christians only too ready and eager to help them along the pathway to elimination.

With the same skills, talents, knowledge, and energy that were the keys to their achievements as Jews, the

National Institute of Allergy and Infectious Diseases, National Institutes of Health, Bethesda, MD 20892

conversos continued their pursuits with the same degrees of success. Furthermore, the problem of competition with the Old Christians did not go away. Rather it was compounded by the fact that there were new undertakings open to the conversos, which previously were denied to them as Jews. Creating New Christians did not diminish competitive disadvantages for less able Old Christians whether in the arena of medicine, banking, public service, trades, or crafts. If anything, adding to the Christian population in equitable fashion only increased longstanding built-in rivalry. Instead of being welcomed into the fold, New Christians continued to face the same old pattern of officially imposed restrictions. Under the guise of holding New Christians suspect of questionable intent, and even infidelity to Christ, the force of physical attack emerged. By the 1440s destructive and murderous riots began in Toledo and Ciudad Real. Greed and the opportunity to rob without legal restrictions exceeded even the religious factor. Once the mobs formed, they could not be controlled.

Persecution of Jews and New Christians had become a way of life, even though antagonism toward New Christians was considered inappropriate by both high levels of State and Church governance. To lessen the agitation and hostility that triggered uncontrollable riots, the government reluctantly agreed to bar Marranos from public posts—a regulation that included official city physicians. Its implementation, however, was defeated by papal nullification on the basis of the fact that such actions involved the persecution of Catholics, regardless of their routes or times of entrance and acceptance into Christianity and the Church. The objectives of hate-inspiring monks and the economic and socially disadvantaged masses were sought by efforts to unmask Marranos as secret Jews through special courts of inquiry. Enlightened and educated Christians, the Popes and the kings, who could not condone injustice and brutality, opposed the Spanish Church's wish to set up and conduct an officially sanctioned Inquisition. Additionally, taking the process beyond papal authority and control, the potential loss of revenues and special avenues of assistance to the monarchies also posed serious considerations. However, the marriage of Isabella to Ferdinand in 1469 provided the critical turning point.

With their subsequent accessions to thrones—Isabella to Castile in 1474 and Ferdinand to Aragon 4 years later—and their joint rule of the unified kingdoms, all sense of humaneness gave way to religious zeal and opportunism. In addition to the confiscated wealth that would come into the royal treasury, the devoutly pious Isabella was personally offended by the traditional Jewish practices of some Marranos on the Passover holiday. In 1480, the King and Queen author-

ized the Spanish Inquisition (Figs. 1 and 2), and its horrors were accepted despite papal objections.

By all means of intrigue and contrivance through spying, witnesses, falsification, trickery, starvation, torture, and forced confessions, the Church inquisitors fiercely sought to bring in evidence and ignored any consideration of creditability or validity. Accusations were equated with guilt, and Marranos were judged and subjected to wide gradations of penalties and punishments. These included penance, restrictions on living and earning circumstances, fines, confiscation of property and personal resources, flogging, hanging, and burning at the stake. Last minute confessions earned the mercy of strangulation for the accused before being put to the fire. Those who successfully escaped capture were burned in effigy, and to satisfy posthumous sentences, remains were dug up and burned in acts symbolic of burning in hell. Sentences were executed at public festivals called Auto-du-Fé (Act of Faith).

Acceptance of Catholicism, in response to the threat and fear of murder based on one's record of birth as a Hebrew, often ended in death as an accused heretic New Christian. Some Marrano families who survived the initial years of horror and managed the process of integration, were completely absorbed into Catholic Spain. Others who were targeted and victimized realized too late that they might well have been better off taking the chance of retaining their faith because the Church had no control or authority over nonconverted Jews. Here again was another link in the connecting chain of ironic tragedies. Even so, the effectiveness and ability of the Spanish clergy and their secular allies to orchestrate trouble and havoc ultimately won out.

Adding to the tragedies were the actions of New Christians who joined in taking on the roles of perse-

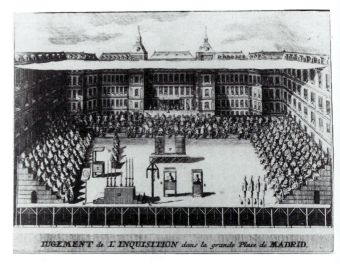

Figure 1. *Depiction of an Inquisition tribunal held in the presence of the King and Queen in Madrid. (Osterreichische Nationalbibliothek, Picture Archives, Vienna.)*

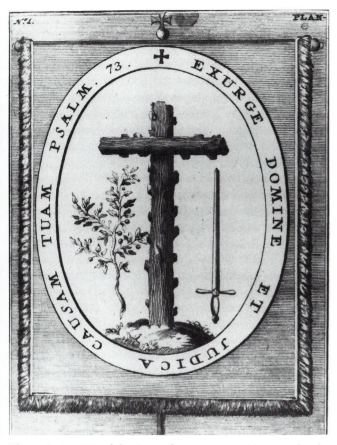

Figure 2. Banner of the Spanish Inquisition. (Osterreichische Nationalbibliothek, Picture Archives, Vienna.)

cutors. Among the fiercest hate mongers and Jew-baiters were some Catholic clergy and monks who had been converted from Judiasm before entering studies for the Church or who were only first or second generation conversos. By exterminating Jewry they hoped to destroy any threatening evidence of their own origins. Even the Grand Inquisitor, the Dominican Tomas de Torquemada, had Jewish ancestry traced to his grandmother who had been a convert. For excessive fanaticism to the point of conjuring up unjustified accusations of heresy involving ecclesiastical dignitaries, he received repeated admonitions from Pope Alexander VI, but even ultimate excommunication did not restrain Torquemada.

Within the New Christian community there were New Christians who found it expedient to preserve their own chances for survival by denouncing fellow conversos, even turning on close family members. Frenzied drives for preservation of self and family that the Inquisitors had brought to tortured minds displaced principles of honesty, integrity, and reason in the human equation. Such acts of perfidy were encouraged, rewarded, and added to the toll. To further the cause of the Inquisition, its perpetrators believed much more

needed to be done if the New Christians were to be completely brought into line and monitored. As long as converts had the opportunity to associate and interact with Jewish counterparts, they were subject to non-Christian influences and their tenuous status could be a continuing problem. There was only one practical solution for the Jewish problem to be brought before the Castile and Aragon rulers. Leaving Spain was the only alternative to accepting conversion.

Because Ferdinand and Isabella realized Spain's continued need to retain the intellectual and economic resources of Jews in critical positions as physicians, financiers, skilled artisans, and government officials, an exodus of Jews from Spain was neither appealing nor to be considered. Additionally, the monarchs were preoccupied with plans for the final elimination of Moslem Spain through the conquest of Granada, the last stronghold of the declining but still troublesome Moors.

On January 2, 1492, Ferdinand's army took Granada. With its fall even more Jews and Moors were added to the Spanish domain and had to be dealt with. Imprisonment, threats, and restrictions alone were not sufficient deterrents as long as there were Jews who, it was believed, could wield influence, corrupt the thinking of New Christians and serve as a source of agitation to the clergy and malcontents. On March 31, 1492, Ferdinand and Isabella were finally persuaded, and they formalized the final solution, an edict to accept either immediate baptism or expulsion. Of the remaining 200,000 Jews, most felt a deep attachment to Spain, because their Spanish heritage traced back to centuries of ancestral residence and contributions to the history of their homeland's glorious culture. Fear and force won many of these for Catholicism. However, their troubles did not end with conversion. While the initial thrust of the Inquisition reached its height in the first 12 years, attacks and executions continued taking a toll beyond the period of expulsion.

For those who chose expulsion there were few options in 1492. A chain reaction of prior European expulsions between 1421 and 1489 had driven Jews out of leading cities of Germany and Italy, e.g., Vienna, Linz, Cologne, Augsburg, Bavaria, Moravia, Perugia, Parma, Milan, and Lucca. Looking elsewhere, in 4 months 100,000 Jews travelled by land to neighboring Portugal and 50,000 set sail for North Africa and Turkey from the designated ports of Cartegena, Valencia, Cadiz, Laredo, Tarragona, and Barcelona.

By indiscriminately sending out Jews as a group to face the turmoil and uncertainties of wandering to find new homes and ways of life, the Spanish monarchs with one swift blow also brought about a cultural and economic rearrangement. The experienced skills and intellects of the Spanish Jews, or Sephardi as they became known (derived from the old name of Spain), would be sown world wide. Losses to Spain, and later Portugal, would become increasingly apparent. True, the confiscated wealth and the considerable financial resources of the banking families remained behind and a new class of Christian artisans and tradesmen developed, but the void of physicians, whether scholars, practitioners, or mentors, would be especially damaging, if not irreparable for centuries to come.

Clergy who evolved through exercises in bigotry worked in concert with noneducated masses who had little opportunity for enlightenment. Joined by others who believed survival and economic advancement could be gained by decimating overshadowing competition, they constituted a formidable antagonist group. That this combination of biased orientation and self-serving motivation would bring the seeds of the Inquisition and expulsion to fruition was understandable, but viewing the royal backgrounds of Ferdinand and Isabella, it is difficult to appreciate that they would serve as the instruments of these inhumane events.

Ferdinand's blood line was not pure Christian; his grandmother was a Jewess. In the liberal ambience of Aragon, his father Juan II's favorable attitude was reflected in the manner with which he honored the Jewish oculist who through surgery restored his eyesight. Isabella seems not to have been influenced to any lasting degree by her half-brother and predecessor Henry IV, who for the 20-year period of his reign, restored a semblance of decency to Castile in contrast to its prior period of turmoil. In the early years of her succession Isabella followed Henry's example of employing a Jewish physician to whom she granted special privileges and exemptions. However, somewhere along the line she found the necessary conditioning to support and sponsor persecution.

PORTUGAL

Portugal shared its early history with that of the other Spanish provinces that constituted the Iberian peninsula. At the end of the 11th century, like Aragon, Castile, Leon, and Navarre, Portugal established itself as a kingdom. Although it remained independent of Spain, common heritage fostered similarity of Spanish and Portuguese languages and cultural development. For the Jews of Portugal, however, there was one fortunate major difference. They enjoyed tranquility and tolerance in scholarly, scientific, and economic pursuits under benevolent Portuguese kings for more than two centuries longer than the Jewish communities of neighboring Spain.

The beneficence of a continuing line of Portuguese monarchs, dating back to the first half of the 13th century, was reflected by the number of Jews who were given high positions of State, and the respect and high regard bestowed upon Jewish physicians. As the pursuit of knowledge by Hebrew scholars was broadly inclusive in medieval Europe, in Portugal, as in Spain, physicians often served royal courts as medical practitioners, astronomers, and astrologers. Under royal patronage they often concurrently served their religious constituencies in appointed high rabbinical posts. In this capacity generations of the distinguished Yahya family served generations of kings, e.g., Pedro (1356–1367), João (1383–1435), and Duarte (1435–1438).

Another distinguished family name in Portuguese medicine was Naverro. The Naverro story began with Moses Naverro, who left Spanish Naverre because of ongoing persecutions. In Portugal, he became physician to King Pedro (1357–1367), Chief Rabbi of Portugal, and Receiver-General of taxes, and he used his good standing with the king to further Jewish causes. Similarly, his grandson Moses Naverro, Chief Rabbi and physician to King João (John) I, played an important role in gaining the protection of his patron. Aware of spreading persecution in Spain, Moses influenced the King to issue a law in 1392 based upon the edicts of Popes Clement VI and Boniface IX, whose bulls forbade forced baptism, beating and robbing Jews, and desecration of Jewish cemeteries. Additionally he obtained the King's protection for Spanish Jews seeking refuge in Portugal.

João, known as a friend and protector of the Jews, paradoxically was responsible for laws restricting them to the ghetto after closing of the gates. Physicians and surgeons were exempt from this restriction, and were permitted to leave if called for an emergency and accompanied by a Christian who carried a light. They also were exempted from the regulation that prohibited entering a Christian home when not accompanied by a Christian.

Under Alfonso V (1438–1458) the Jews once again enjoyed the comforts and security of restored freedom and tranquility and the benefits of cultural and economic pursuits, which for them translated into prosperity. It was Alfonso's reign that produced the distinguished scholar and statesman Isaac Abravanel, who had succeeded his father as Royal Treasurer, and the highly regarded court physician, Ephraim ben Sancho. Unfortunately, regardless of Alfonso's favor, Ephraim fell victim to court jealousies and intrigues and left Portugal to continue medical practice in Turkey. Upon arrival in Constantinople Ephraim was welcomed and honored by Sultan Mahmud II the Great, in whose court he again enjoyed favor in the position of personal physician.

Similarly Abravanel was forced to flee the Portuguese court for Castile because of his friendship with the Duke of Braganza who had been condemned to death by

King João II, successor to Alfonso. In Spain Abranavel rendered great service to Ferdinand and Isabella in the management of personal and State finances until his second exile. His plea to the monarchs to rescind the expulsion edict for Jews, even when supplemented by a substantial offer of gold, failed. Once again religious zeal and visions of personal gain won out over logic, indebtedness, and morality. Although Abravanel's royal patrons afforded him the opportunity to remain in Spain and maintain his Jewish status, he refused the offer of privileged exception. Joining the exiled Jewish community, he went to Naples.

With Alfonso's death in 1458 Portugal's role in the Golden Age also faded away. The long arm of the Spanish Christian monarchs reached out to involve Alfonso's successors, João II (1487–1495) and Manoel I (1495–1521) in dispensing comparable bigotry and persecution.

João II began his reign with continuing appreciation and employment of Jewish physicians. Their contributions to mathematics and astronomy were prominent in Portugal's role in the age of discovery and exploration and in furthering Columbus' cause. Abraham Zacuto (1450–1525) of the faculties of Salamanca and Saragossa, fled from Spain in the expulsion of 1492, and received court appointments upon arriving in Portugal, first with João, then Manoel. The original information given in Zacuto's classic astronomy treatise *Almanach Perpetuum*, data derived from his astronomical tables, and use of his astrolabes proved seminal as navigational aides. These aides guided Portuguese explorations, including Vasco da Gama's historical voyage around the Cape of Good Hope to the East Indies.

Another Jewish physician, Joseph Vecinho, was a member of the King's commission appointed to examine and judge Columbus' proposal to João. Vecinho had translated Zacuto's treatise from Hebrew to Latin and Spanish and gave a copy to Columbus. His improved designs of navigational instruments were key factors in the charting of Columbus' course.

Unfortunately, in 1492 João looked away from his trusted and valued Jewish physicians and aides, and looked toward opportunism arising out of the disastrous Spanish expulsion. The only Jews he allowed to enter Portugal were either wealthy enough to afford a steep charge or were skilled artisans who could work in the production of munitions. For a lesser sum financially limited Jews could stay a few months while searching for a subsequent new home. In João's practical realm, economic gain superseded compassion, and there wasn't any place in Portugal for those too poor to pay. Even so his promises were not fulfilled for the few hundred thousand who were granted temporary admission. Upon arrival in Lisbon they not only were ordered to leave; the promised ships to aid their departures were insufficient and grossly inadequate, regardless of the huge sums unscrupulous owners charged for charters.

Upon succeeding João, Manoel initially was favorably influenced by Zacuto to be sympathetic to the Jewish plight and mindful of the role of Jewish subjects in Portugal's state of prosperity. However, Isabella and Ferdinand had other ideas, and higher in Manoel's priority was the ambitious possibility of becoming ultimate heir to the Spanish throne through marriage to their daughter, the young Princess Isabella. Isabella and Ferdinand refused consent for the marriage of their daughter to Manoel unless Portugal also eliminated nonChristians. In compliance, Manoel upon the signing of his marriage contract with Isabella in 1496, issued orders for the expulsion of Jews. The only alternative was death and confiscation of the condemned's property. Even his esteemed physician-astronomer Abraham Zacuto once again was forced to depart his country, but this second exile would not be his last. After reaching Tunis, Zacuto lived there until arrival of the invading Spaniards forced another flight and a third refuge in Turkey.

Like Ferdinand and Isabella, Manoel wanted to accomplish more than just expulsion; he sought the creation of New Christians. He ordered forced baptism of Jewish children, expecting that parents might be willing to accept conversion as an alternative to expulsion. They then could remain as a family. Also by delaying forced departures until after the announced expulsion date he forced Jews to listen to conversion preaching, while simultaneously depriving the listeners food and water. When all else failed the captive Jews were forced into involuntary conversion regardless of their wishes or resistance. Of 20,000 Jews subjected to these physically and emotionally torturous schemes, very few escaped. Others were given to grandees as slaves. Some elected suicide by jumping into the waters of the harbor. Many, however, accepted baptism rather than face the frustrations of further wandering, dangerous travel by leaky vessels, and the chances of being taken to Arab countries for sale into slavery or being captured at sea by pirates and held for ransom.

As in Spain, compulsory baptisms did not accomplish their objective. In Portugal, Marranos continued to practice Judaic precepts in secret. Others, despite hardships and obstacles, managed to leave for countries where they were free to revert to their birth-endowed faith. To check this exodus, Manoel prohibited further departures without official permission. Again as in Spain, Old Christians were angered, and with escalating hate pitted themselves against New Christians. A Dominican inspired massacre in Lisbon followed in 1506. The next year Manoel allowed Marranos to leave the country, but in 1521 restrictions again were reinstituted. In opposition to zealots' urgings to set up an Inquisition, Pope Alexander pointed out the lack of wisdom and purpose in compelling adherence to a religion into which one was forced. Nevertheless under the papal authority of Clement VII, King João III (1521–1557) brought the Inquisition to Portugal in 1531. As in Spain, the toll of Marranos who met their fates at Auto-da-Fés included leaders of Portuguese medicine.

AFTERMATH

"Fanatic fools, that in those twilight times, With wild religion cloaked the worst of crimes."
John Langhorne, *The Country Justice*, Part III, Line 122 (1777)

Although Spain and Portugal followed different sequences in pathways of attack, each accomplished the identical objective. In the transitional years between medieval times and the Renaissance, Judaism was eradicated within each country's respective domain. Spain's attack was a gradual, orchestrated process that covered 100 years. The pogroms of 1391 were followed by a series of progressively weakening and eroding attacks. Repressive laws, periodic riots and massacres, persecution, torture, and conversions to Catholicism, induced by tactics of fear and life-threatening panic, culminated in the expulsion of 1492.

Portugal's attack was speedy and required only the year of 1497 to accomplish Judaism's nationwide near extinction through simultaneous expulsion and forced mass baptisms. In 39 years the destruction of whatever remained of Judaism in the conversos began. Despite biases against New Christian status, some Portuguese conversos had continued to rise to high echelons of medicine, government, finance, and commerce. However, in 1536 with the institution of a papal sanctioned Inquisition, even the cloak of religious conversion offered little if any security.

In contrast to diminishing intensity of the postexpulsion Spanish Inquisition in the mid 16th century, the Portuguese counterpart proceeded with even greater ferocity and terror. When Portugal joined Spain in 1580 in a union that lasted for 88 years, the gates were opened for Portuguese conversos to look to Spain for better socioeconomic conditions and respite from the severity of their Portuguese persecution. But as soon as the possibility of removing some legal, if not social, distinctions between New and Old Christians was finding spokesmen in the Spanish Church, the large influxes of Portuguese Marranos into Spain set a hostile backlash in motion. Perception of Judaizers in the Christian mix reactivated the earlier frenzied tempo of the Spanish Inquisition. Auto-da-Fés continued in unabated fashion in Portugal until 1739 and in Spain until 1790.

The most intellectually desirable and demonstrably contributing members of Spanish-Portuguese society, including physicians and scientific scholars, were not spared. Whatever reasonable thought might have motivated the drive to accomplish religious conversions was lost sight of in the blindness of zealous implementation. The mentality of the hate-mongers could not allow for even the practicality of availing themselves of the special skills of Marrano physicians. The need to perpetuate the disdained image of a genetically marked Jew regardless of his new religion took precedence. The propagated myth that Jewish physicians and druggists deliberately poisoned their patients was expanded to incriminate New Christians. Forced confessions obtained under torture added many in the class of healers to the numbers burned at the stake. If ever there was a goal to consolidate and transfer the magnificent fruits of a Moslem-Judaic-Christian culture to a singular Catholic entity, any possibility of integration gave way to the fanaticism of self-defeating laws, governance, and Church guidance.

Despite the objective of missionary conversion efforts, the 1449 discriminatory edicts of the Council of Toledo served to perpetuate intrinsic resentment against Jews who had assumed christianity. According to the statute of "limpieza de sangra" (purity of blood) anyone of Jewish or Moorish ancestry was barred from holding office or receiving titles or honors. Initially there was sufficient opposition from the King, the Pope, higher clergy, and statesmen to generate a lack of acceptance and enforcement of edicts of this nature against New Christians.

With the expulsions from Spain in 1492 and Portugal in 1497, legal restrictions formulated against professing Jews became academic. When continuing resentment against the Jewish presence was expanded to include conversos, New Christians became primary targets despite the fact that their assumption of a new religious status was of their oppressors' doing. Then in 1501, in Granada the Catholic monarchs signed a decree that required pure Catholic blood for anyone to engage in social practices, which included the work of physicians and surgeons.

Since common religious faith could no longer be an acceptable factor, ethnicity through a blood line would henceforth serve as the critical differentiating criterion to satisfy discontented and bigoted countrymen. Apparently, however, specific applications of this law were being ignored as most practicing Iberian physicians and apothecaries in the 16th century could still be traced to Jewish origins. Many Jewish converts sought to enter the practice of medicine despite the great danger they subjected themselves to in rendering this service. With even the slightest trace of Marrano or Morisco (Moorish convert) blood, any found guilty of even a minor misdemeanor would be subject to full theologic and social prejudice. Convictions for accused heresy incurred penalties to be assumed by successive generations of descendents of those sentenced.

Because of the names they made for themselves and the famed reputations gained by Jewish physicians,

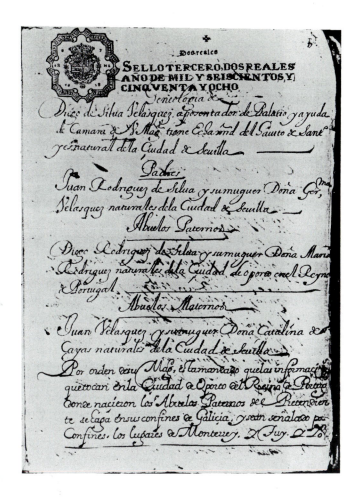
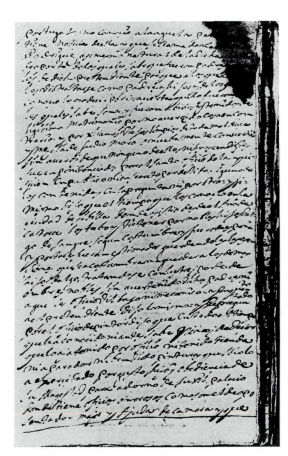

Figure 3. Limpieza de sangre for Velasquez, 1658; certifying to his Old Christian parentage without taint by ancestors from bad races, Jews, Moors, or recent converts. (From Weisenthal S. Sails of Hope).

exemptions commonly were granted to Marrano practitioners. In his 1594 treatise *Examen de Ingenios*, a Madrid physician named Juan Huarte de Juan explained justification for the policy of exemptions by correlating special qualities of the Jewish race with the particular talents required for the practice of medicine. For historical evidence of inborn character that was supposedly formed hundreds of years previously, Huarte referred to factors associated with 40 years of Jewish wandering during the exodus from Egypt to Palestine. Dietary manna and exposure to desert environment and hot climate, he theorized, served as *in utero* determinants for the development of high degrees of intelligence. At the same time Huarte indicated that these endowed Jewish children had black bile that made them cunning and sly and hostile to all other religious faiths. Against this background was a curious view that associated dishonor with the profession of physician, largely because so many of its practitioners were New Christians. Since expression of contempt for and aviodance of anything that suggested Judiasm were consid-

ered to be demonstrations of pure Christian descent, science and medicine were looked upon as unattractive pursuits. As a result medical endeavor was replaced by a vacuum.

Despite the usual opposition of the more enlightened Spanish segment, a new statute promulgated in Toledo in 1547 gained official approval by Pope Paul VI and King Philip II in 1555. From that point on "limpieza de sangre"—freedom from Jewish or Moorish blood—became an official requirement for medical practice (Fig. 3). Even Moor and Morisco physicians who remained in Granada came under the same restrictions and harassments. It was ironic that the culture that had contributed so much to the development of medicine could now pursue its practice only illegally. In 1609, 117 years after expulsion of their former Jewish colleagues, the same fate befell Morisco practitioners.

By the 17th century multiple exclusionary statutes covered a large group of medical, military, judiciary, religious, academic, governmental, and fraternal endeavors. It was not until some 300 years later, in 1885, that the legal obligation of proving absence of antecedent trait of Moorish, Jewish, or otherwise heretic or infidel tainted blood was abolished.

The expulsion of the Jews, compounded by the Inquisition's toll and its Auto-da-Fés, reduced Spain's and Portugal's physician populations to the point of producing self-inflicted problems in public health for several municipalities. Shortages of physicians required to render personal services occurred in principal cities, and a shortage of university medical professors occurred. Enforcement of limpieza de sangre laws added to both the acuteness of this situation and the motivation of converso physicians to undertake the hardships of leaving homes to seek distant tolerant and hospitable worksites. In rural areas, the anti-Semitic havoc provoked by low clergy and the ill-educated masses further contributed to the lack of skilled physicians. Health care necessarily was left to empiric and superstitious practices, astrologers, and conjurers of magic.

A mark of the effect of physician and surgeon shortages was its impact on Spain's regulation of medical practices. From the time of Alfonso V, Aragon had a tribunal to examine practitioners and screen out the incompetent and illy prepared. This body became known as the Promedicato, named after the king's first physician, or promedico, who served as a member. With unification of Aragon and Castile in 1477, a central Promedicato was established and empowered to license physicians, surgeons, midwives, apothecaries, and spice merchants. Also given judicial authority, the composition of the Promedicato was broadened to include physicians, auditors, magistrates, law enforcement officers, and a member of the judiciary.

Coming under the Promedicato's purview were distinct classes within the university trained group: (1) holders of doctoral degrees who were oriented to university careers; (2) liceniado (licentiate) and bachiller (bachelor) medical graduates who held medical degrees, but who did not elect to undertake required formalities for the doctorate; and (3) Latin surgeons, university trained, in contrast to Romance Surgeons who were meagerly trained in apprenticeships. By the 16th century higher standards were in place. Surgeons and apothecaries were required to have 4 years of minimum training as apprentices before meeting eligibility for examination, and physicians' examinations included practical demonstrations of diagnostic and therapeutic competency in the handling of hospital patients.

Loss of the major segment of physicians resulting from expulsion of the Jews and Moors and exclusion of Marranos and Moriscos apparently could be compensated for only by lowering competency standards. Under Philip II in 1567, midwives and grocery dealers in spices and aromatic drugs were removed from the purview of the Protomedicato. In 1588 authorization was given to license practitioners of a single empiric

procedure as long as the procedure was carried out in consultation with licensed surgeons—e.g., the algebrista set bones, the hermista reduced hernias, the sacador de la piedra removed bladder stones, the batidor de la catarata couched cataracts, and the sacamuela extracted teeth. With progressive shortages, in 1603 Philip III gave legal status even to Romance surgeons who had 2 years experience as an apprentice to a physician or master surgeon and 3 years of additional hospital experience.

The regulatory and discriminatory practices of Spain were extended to its newly founded and conquered lands. As a result severe health care shortages of crisis proportions were wrought in central and southern Mexico (known as "New Spain"). The appointment of a Protomedico in 1525 was aimed at protecting residents from the influx of irregular healers into Mexico City who were responsible for more harm than healing. Working to an opposite end, royal orders received in 1535 required enforcement of a limpieza de sangre policy. These diminished whatever chance there was for university training of, or care by, competent physicians of Jewish or Moorish descent or possible assistance from native Aztec healers. Consequently, by 1545 there were only four Protomedicato certified physicians in Mexico City. Of these, one was in ill health, one was in jail suspected of sorcery, and a third was unable to produce a valid diploma and was experiencing legal difficulties.

In orchestrating its own cultural decline and dissipation of its Golden Age, Renaissance Spain suffered irreversible regression of its preeminent position in the development of science and medicine. Through their self-inflicted losses, Spain and Portugal indirectly and unintentionally contributed to advancements in other countries. Human values that formerly had taken root and been nurtured in the Iberian milieu were seeded elsewhere. With forced emigration many eminent physicians seeking refuge found opportunities to transplant careers and contribute to health care and the pioneering of medicine, particularly in Turkey, Italy, the Netherlands, North Africa, England, and Hamburg, Germany. Other physicians moved to the Spanish and Portuguese new possessions.

In the history of medicine in these countries, many physicians who distinguished themselves, especially by contributing to the literature and through original findings and descriptions, can be traced to Spanish-Portuguese origins. Safe entrenchment and opportunities for Jews and reverted Marranos to openly follow religious practices, however, did not always ensure permanency of resettlement. Unexpected waves of periodic persecution and expulsion from newly found homes continued the pattern of recurrent uprooting and resettlement. Thus in Jewish and Marrano genealogic trees, medical graduates of eminent Spanish and Portuguese universities and their physician descendants were found widespread throughout European, middle eastern, and colonial countries. Common heritages were reflected in family names such as Acosta, Bueno, Cardosa, de Castro, Mendes, Rodriguez, Sanchez, and da Silva. Other examples include the da Fonseca and Nunez medical families who were linked by 20 geographically dispersed members. A spectrum of varied experiences can be seen in the representative accounts, excerpted from Kagan and from Friedenwald, that follow.

BIBLIOGRAPHY

Dale PM. Medical Biographies, the Ailments of Thirty-three Famous Persons. Norman, Oklahoma: University of Oklahoma Press, 1952, pp. 16–19.

Encyclopedia Judaica. Jerusalem: Keter Publishing House, Vol 11, Medicine, 1971, pp. 1178–1196.

Friedenwald H. The Jews and Medicine, Essays. Baltimore: Johns Hopkins Press, 1944.

Fuson RH. The Log of Christopher Columbus (translation). Camden, ME: International Marine Publishing Co., 1987.

Grangel LS, Palermo JR. Medicina y sociedad en la espana renacentista. In: Entralgo PL (ed.) Historia Universal de la Medicina. Barcelona: Salvat Editores, 1973, pp. 181–189.

Grayzel S. A History of the Jews. Philadelphia: Jewish Publication Society, 1968.

Hordes S. The inquisition and the Crypto-Jewish community in colonial New Spain. In: Perry MD, Cruz A (eds.) Cultural Encounters: The Impact of the Inquisition in Spain and the New World. Berkeley, CA: University of California Press, 1991.

Hordes S. The inquisition and the Crypto-Jewish community in New Spain and New Mexico. In: Perry, ME, Cruz A (eds.) Op. Cit., pp. 207–217.

Johnson P. A History of the Jews. New York: Harper and Row, 1987.

Kagan SR. Jewish Contributions to Medicine in America. Boston: Boston Medical Publishing Company, 1939.

Kagan SR. Jewish Medicine. Boston: Medico-Historical Press, 1952.

Kayserling M. Christopher Columbus and the Participation of the Jews in the Spanish and Portugese Discoveries (translated by Gross C), 4th ed. New York: Hermon Press, 1968.

Kayserling M. Sephardim, Romanische Possien der Juden in Spanien. Leipzig, 1859.

Perry ME, Cruz AJ, eds. Cultural Encounters, The Impact of the Inquisition in Spain and the New World. Berkeley, CA: University of California Press, 1991.

Preuss J. Biblical and Talmudic Medicine (translated and edited by Rosner F). New York: Sanhedrin Press, 1978.

Rise GR. Medicine in New Spain. In: Numbers RL (ed.) Medicine in the New World. Knoxville:University of Tennessee Press, 1987, pp. 12–63.

Sokoloff L. Rise and decline of Jewish quota in medical school admissions. Bull NY Acad Med, 68: 497–518, 1992

Wiesenthal S. Sails of Hope: The Secret Mission of Christopher Columbus (translated by Winston C, Winston R). New York: Macmillan, 1973.

Yerushalmi YH. From Spanish court to Italian ghetto. In: Isaac Cardoso: A Study in Seventeenth Century Marranism and Jewish Apologetics. New York: Columbia University Press, 1971. □

Spain, Portugal, Christopher Columbus, and the Jewish Physician: Spanish-Portuguese Physicians in the Diaspora

Sheldon G. Cohen, M.D.

"I have learned . . . toleration from the intolerant, and kindness from the unkind; yet strange I am ungrateful to those teachers."

Kahlil Gibran
Sand and Foam, 1926

SPANISH—PORTUGUESE PHYSICIANS IN THE DIASPORA

Turkey

The Moslem capture of Constantinople in 1453 would again offer a favorable setting for Jewish physicians to seek and take up opportunities that began to fade with the Moors' loss of Spain. Thanks to Islamic respect for cultural and scientific pursuits, unrestricted practices of medicine could be resumed for Spanish and Portuguese exiles fortunate enough to reach Turkey. The Turkish populace along with the ruling sultans, emirs, and pashas had come to value the medical skills, knowledge, and ethical standards they came to identify with the new Spanish and Portuguese immigrants. Here again, preferred Jewish physicians were favored over their Christian and Moslem counterparts.

Initially the way to Turkey was paved in the late 15th century by Ephraim ben Sancho who, until falling a victim to intrigue in Portugal's royal court, had been Alphonso V's favorite physician. On reaching Constantinople, Ephraim became personal physician to the Sul-tan Mahmud II the Great. The tradition in medicine then passed on to his son Abraham, who also was a poet.

Then there was Joseph Hamon who found himself faced with exile from Granada at an advanced age. His family name was well known and highly regarded in medicine in Granada, Isaac Hamon having established himself as a physician favored in the court of the king. But as Granada fell, Joseph was subjected to continuing Spanish persecution. Invited to Constantinople by the Sultan, he served as personal physician first to Byazid II (1481–1512) and later Selin I. Thereafter for almost a century, Hamon family members continued the tradition beginning with Joseph's son, Moses (c. 1490–1565) as physician to Sultan Solaiman I, and in turn Moses' son, Joseph II, served Solaiman's son, Selin II (1566–1574).

Among historical notables for whom Turkey provided an ultimate refuge was Abraham ben Samuel Zacutus/Zacuto (1452–1525) (Fig. 4), the scholar physician, historian, and astronomer whose navigational aids guided Christopher Columbus' and Vasco da Gama's voyages of discovery. Fleeing first from Portugal, then Tunis, Zacutus reached Turkey in the early years of the 16th century and died in Damascus.

Juan Rodrigo De Castelbranco, also known as Amatus Lusitanus (1511–1568) (Fig. 5), was considered the outstanding clinician and medical botanist of his day. Fleeing the impending Portuguese Inquisition, he began a series of wanderings, first practicing in Antwerp. Next, in Italy he became Professor of Medicine at Ferrara (1540–1577) from where he was called to Rome to treat Pope Julius III. With the advent of yet another Inquis-

National Institute of Allergy and Infectious Diseases, National Institutes of Health, Bethesda, MD 20892

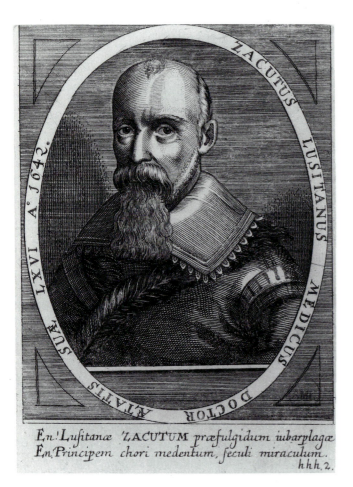

Figure 4. *Abraham Zacutus (1452–1525); taken from an engraving (courtesy of the National Library of Medicine).*

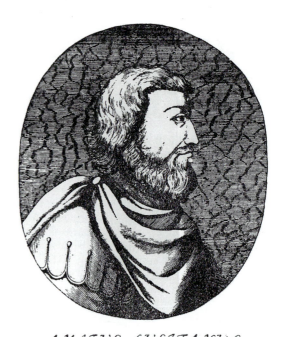

AMATUS LUSITANUS

En Arzt von Castelblanco einer Stadt in Portugall gebürtig, hies eigentlich Johannes Rodriguer de Castelblanco, lebte in der Mitte des 16 Jahrhunderts, und bekante sich zu Thessalonich zur Jüdischen Religion.

Figure 5. *Amatus Lusitanus (1511–1568), taken from an engraving; in* Friedenwald H. The Jews and Medicine (*courtesy of Johns Hopkins University Press).*

ition in Ancona, Amatus fled once again to reach Salonika.

Daniel de Fonseca (b. 1677) was baptized at 8 years of age and entered the priesthood. Secretly returning to Judaism, he fled to France where he studied medicine, then he went on to Turkey. Subsequently spending some intervening years as physician and advisor to the reigning prince at Bucharest, he returned to Turkey as physician to Sultan Ahmad III. After the Sultan's deposition, he returned to France. In Paris, Fonseca associated with Voltaire who referred to him as a learned and talented man and perhaps the only philosopher among the Jews of his time.

Italy

Italy long had been appreciated for its history of favorable treatment of Jewish communities and of Italian Jewish physicians who enjoyed a tradition of serving nobles and popes. In 1498 when the Jews were expelled from Provence, Bonnet de Lattes (d. 1515) went to Rome, and became physician to successive Popes, Alexander VI and Leo X. Simultaneously he held the positions of Judge of the highest Court of Appeals and Chief Rabbi of Rome.

As nonecclesiastic schools, Padua and Perugio were among the few medical faculties, with Montpellier and Salamanca, that admitted Jewish students. It thus followed quite naturally that fleeing Spanish-Portuguese victims of the Inquisition and expulsion would seek Italy as a safe and desirable haven.

Among these was Joseph Vecinho, whose navigational aids and translation of Zacutus' astronomical *Almanac* aided the explorations of Christopher Columbus and Vasco da Gama. Vecinho initially settled in Ferrara then later in Venice, where his grandson Abraham Vecinho continued the family heritage and tradition of physician and astronomer.

Judah Abravanel was the son of Isaac Abravanel whose financial skills and resources for the Spanish Court were so highly prized by Ferdinand and Isabella. As a child Judah was kidnapped and brought up as a Christian by the Church in Portugal while his family was seeking refuge in Naples, Genoa, and Venice. Later he escaped and after joining his father, gained distinction as a physician and author of scholarly works.

Isaac's brother, Joseph, also a physician and scholar, gained a considerable reputation in Venice and Ferrara.

Philotheo Elia Montalto, after fleeing Portugal and reaching Florence in 1606, became physician to Grand Duke Frederick. He was renown for original work on vision and nervous and mental diseases. In 1611 he left for France at the urging of the Queen Marie de Medici to become her personal physician.

Jacob Mantino (1490-1549), brought to Italy as a child, studied medicine and philosophy at Bologna and Padua. He was noted for translations of classic works of Moslem physicians from Hebrew to Latin, and he also served as a rabbi, court physician to Pope Paul III, and Professor of Medicine at the University of Rome.

Curiously the tolerant environment of Italy fluctuated in problematic fashion and varied from time to time and from region to region. Periodic leniency often alternated with periodic persecution and restrictions. Following the influx of Spanish-Portuguese immigrants during the first half of the 16th century, expulsions were ordered in Venice and Naples. Jews were also excluded from the central Italian Papal state, except for Rome and Ancona where large contributions to the Papal treasury were derived from Jewish taxpayers. However, quite the opposite, northern Italy remained open.

In other extremes of Papal variability, Engenius IV, Nicholas V, and Calixtus III, in concert with temporal sovereigns, promulgated antiJewish decrees. Yet at the same time they employed personal Jewish physicians. On one hand there was Paul III's (1534-1539) encouragement of Jewish settlers who in 1534 had been expelled from Naples and in 1540 he openly accepted Marranos promising them protection from the Inquisition. The same policy was continued by Paul's successor Julius III until Cardinal Caraffa, who had been a Grand Inquisitor, assumed the Papacy in 1555. In an abrupt reversal of humanism he followed two different courses. First, he instituted the Venetian "solution" of segregation in Rome, where he created a Ghetto on one bank of the Tiber river. More fiercely in Ancona he sought out Marranos for burning at-the-stake.

Whereas Pius IV had a Jewish physician, David de Pomis (b. 1525), author of *De Medico Hebres Enarratio Apoligica* (a scholarly defense of the Jewish physician), Pius V (1566-1572) was relentless in the exercise of his antiSemitic influence. He expelled Italian Jewish communities, some whose existences dated back to antiquity. Nevertheless, the overall prospect of hope and promise continued to bring physician exiles and escapees to Italy. Of these, several family names remained prominent in medicine for many generations thereafter.

Jacob Hebraeus Rosales (1588-1662) was a Portuguese physician, mathematician, astrologer, poet, and author of literary works. He conducted a distinguished medical practice that included the Archbishop of Braga and the Duke of Braganca, the house that subsequently took over the rule of Portugal in 1640. After reaching Rome in 1625, Rosales devoted himself to pursuits in mathematics and astrology which brought him into personal contact and scientific interactions with Galileo.

Rodriguez de Fonseca (b. mid 16th century) became Professor of Medicine successively at Pisa and Padua (1615-1622). He was recognized for varied work—the renewal of ancient medical classics, commentaries on Hippocrates, and treatises on internal diseases, fevers, surgery, and pharmaceutics. His son, Gabriel, also taught at Pisa; he then became Professor of Medicine at Rome. He was physician successively to three Popes—Gregory XV (1621-1623), Urban VIII (1623-1644), and Innocent X (1644-1655), and was author of several medical treatises including *Medici Oeconomia*.

Fernando Cardosa (1610-1680), after attaining the position of court physician to King Philip IV, left Madrid for Venice where he changed his name to Isaac and reverted to Judaism. Later settling in Verona, he was greatly honored by both Christians and Jews as a learned physician and celebrated as an author. His work included an extensive treatise that encompassed cosmography, physics, medicine, philosophy, theology, and natural science *Las Excellencias y Calunias de los Hebros*, a defense of the Jewish faith. A brother, Miguel (1630-1703), migrated to Venice with him and also returned to Judaism. Miguel practiced medicine in Leghorn, became physician to the Bey of Tripoli, and ultimately in Cairo, became physician to the Pasha of Egypt.

The de Castro family of physicians took up practices in Antwerp, Hamburg, Denmark, France, Holland, and England. Stephen Rodrigo de Castro (b. 1559) became a distinguished Professor of Medicine at Pisa and also was a gifted poet, historian, and expert on social sciences. His contemporary Zacutus Lusitanus spoke of him as the Phoenix of Medicine. Stephen was one of Italy's outstanding clinicians; his publications on pleuritis, tympanism, and epilepsy were widely known and frequently cited.

The curious popularity of Jewish physicians in Italy, in the face of unpredictable episodes of hostility, restrictions, and attacks, has been viewed in the light of a number of characteristics of that period. Pertinent was a combination of factors—Christian superstitious belief in the actuality of Jewish possession of magic arts and the Jewish physicians' unselfish demonstrations of dedication to their healing mission. Compounding these was a recognized and keenly felt shortage of Christian medical practitioners.

Holland

In the early history of the Netherlands, its few Jewish settlers had been victims of hostility and had suffered periodic expulsions from some provinces and cities. They were subjected to expressions of hatred in the country's Catholic oriented literature, restrictions on movements and occupations, and acts of persecution. In the kingdom's later evolution to the independent state of Holland, exiled Jewish physicians would find another safe and welcome shelter. However, this opportunity did not occur until the Dutch too had experienced and freed themselves from Spanish oppression.

In 1477 the marriage of Mary of Burgundy to Archduke Maximillian, the son of Emperor Frederick IV, resulted in union of the Netherlands with Austria and as a consequence its passing to the Spanish crown as a possession. At the time of the beginning of the Spanish Inquisition and expulsion of 1492, Holland, as a province of Spain, provided a practical way-station for Marranos who secretly were attempting to move on to Italy and Turkey.

Resentment against the Spanish under the fanatic rule of Philip II was compounded by the Church's domination and Catholic efforts to eliminate Protestantism, which then was taking root. Attempts to institute the Inquisition in Holland added impetus to the Dutch struggle for independence under William of Orange. Victory for the Dutch in 1581 eventuated in creation of a refuge of freedom and escape from Spain and Portugal. Between 1604 and 1605, Jews were granted charters in Alkamaar, Rotterdam, and Haarlem, and Marranos were permitted to openly practice Judaism. Holland no longer was just a temporary stopping-off point. The port city of Amsterdam evolved into a thriving community and then developed into a center of world trade. Portuguese Marrano-Jewish skills and intellectual resources contributed to Holland's growth in commerce and finance and in development of silk, tobacco, diamond, sugar, and book printing industries.

Especially important in this socio-cultural climate was Jewish involvement in medical practice. The Jewish physicians of Holland achieved considerable reputations for clinical excellence.

Abravanel and Zacuto were among familiar family names of Jewish physicians who reached Amsterdam. Joseph II (d. 1620) and Samuel Abravanel (d. 1621) were descendants of Isaac Abravanel, who is remembered as Ferdinand and Isabella's financial minister. Abraham Zacuto, physician and astronomer, who designed Christopher Columbus' navigational aids, was represented by his great-grandson Abraham Zacutus Lusitanus (1575–1642). He was famed as an anatomist, pathologist, clinician, and therapeutist. His 12 volume *De Medicorum Principum Historia* was the first work to deal with the history of medicine and his code of ethics for physicians became widely known. He wrote on plague, diphtheria, eruptive fevers, and malignant

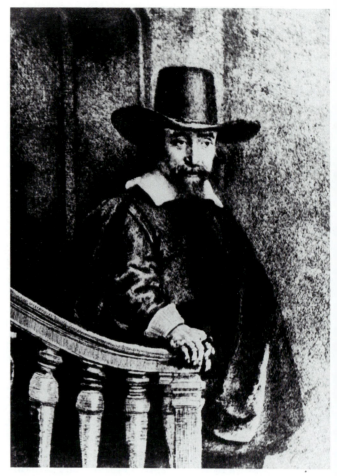

Figure 6. *Ephraim Hezekiah Bueno (?-1665), portrait by Rembrandt (courtesy of the National Library of Medicine).*

growths and provided the original description of alcaptonuria.

Of the Bueno family physician-scholar network, in Amsterdam alone during the mid-late 1600's there were no less than eight members. Two were especially recorded in history. Joseph Bueno in 1625 was called to the sickbed of Prince Maurits of Orange and his son Ephraim Hezekiah's portrait by Rembrandt (Fig. 6) is in the Rijs Museum collection.

Benjamin Mussafia (1606–1675) was distinguished as a physician, philologist, and scholar. He practiced successively in Hamburg and Blueckstadt and became physician to King Christian IV of Denmark. After the King's death, Mussafia settled in Amsterdam where he practiced medicine and joined the College of Rabbis. Among his several books was *Sacro-Medicae Sententiae ex Bibliis*, the earliest work by a physician on Biblical medicine.

Of the da Silva family of physicians, the literary accomplishments of two of its Amsterdam members were noteworthy. Samuel da Silva in 1623 published a book attacking the philosopher Uriel da Costa's view

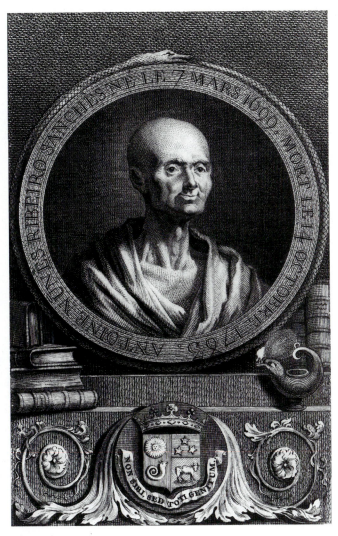

Figure 7. Antonio Rebeiro Sanchez (1699–1783) (Courtesy of the National Library of Medicine).

on immortality. Zachariah da Silva edited *Schola Salernitana* and in 1648 edited William Harvey's work, which subsequently was translated into the English *Anatomical Exercises Concerning the Motion of the Heart and Blood.*

Vincente (Isaac) de Roccomora (1600–1684), a Spanish Marrano, was educated for the Church. As a Cominican monk he was confessor to the Infanta Maria, who subsequently became Empress of Austria. At age 43, de Roccomora fled to Amsterdam, studied medicine and joined the Jewish Community actively engaging in its endeavors.

Antonio Ribeira Sanchez (1699–1783) (Fig. 7), after reaching Holland, studied medicine at Leyden under the famous Dutch physician Herman Boerhaave. Upon Boerhaave's recommendation, Sanchez in 1740 was invited to Russia as personal physician to Ivan Antonovich. As a very successful and highly regarded physician in St. Petersburg, he was elected to the Imperial Academy of Science and successively served in the courts of the Empresses Elizabeth and Catherine II. However, his fortunes turned in 1757 when he was ordered to resign and leave the country, having incurred the disfavor of Catherine for professing Judaism. Sanchez spent the rest of his life in Paris as an eminent physician dedicating his services to the poor. He was recognized for his work on syphilis, which included publication of scientific papers and the introduction of treatment with sublimate of mercury.

A unique note in Holland's story was its considerate reception of the Jewish physician, whether during or after life. In the previous account of Italy, reference was made to Philotheus Eliajus Montalto, a professing Jew from Portugal who became physician to the Grand Duke of Florence. In seeking Montalto as her personal physician, the French Queen Marie de Medici obtained special Church dispensation and once in the country insured a protected and favored role for him in her court. After Montalto's death in 1611, the Queen, having held him in such high regard, ordered his body taken to Amsterdam for a religious burial service and interment in a Jewish cemetery. Neither then was possible in France.

Antwerp

There is evidence that as early as the 14th century a few Jews had resided in Antwerp. More definitely in 1480 local authorities obtained a charter permitting Jews to settle in Antwerp upon condition that they not give reason for scandal. Next, in 1536 the Holy Roman Emperor Charles V of the Spanish and Hapsburg Empire issued an order of safe conduct for Portuguese New Christians which enabled Marranos to live, acquire homes, and engage in business in the Flemish settlement.

Two important factors provided incentives for immigration to Antwerp. First, the port had become the commercial center of Portuguese East Indian trade and thus the site of branches of wealthy Lisbon merchant and banking houses. Second, the magistrates were moved by a spirit of tolerance. Marranos both prospered in Antwerp and were spared from the Inquisition which had not been authorized in the Low Countries although they were under Spanish rule.

A number of other factors, however, combined to generate threatening agitation against Antwerp's Marranos. First, there was the paradoxical circumstance of secret Jews enjoying privileges under a Catholic prince. Compounding this source of hostility, wealthy Marranos were using the Spanish Netherlands as base of transit to escape to Moslem countries. Furthermore, they were suspected of aiding the escalating Protestant Reformation as another means of escape from the Catholic Church. Ultimately, the sovereigns were influenced to revise their attitude to the Marranos.

Over the objections of city officials, an imperial decree in 1545 ordered all Marranos who had come from Portugal before 1543 to leave Antwerp. Despite the municipality's unwillingness to enforce orders and their attempts to keep secret Jews among them, the decree was reissued in 1549. Most of the Marrano families then were forced to depart. Only those who had resided in Antwerp for the previous 6 years and who had promised to strictly adhere to Catholicism's demands were allowed to remain but they were not given protective rights of domicile.

During this early 16th century period of relative tranquility in the Spanish Netherlands, Antwerp, like Amsterdam, played host to fleeing Marrano physicians. Among the especially prominent was Amatus Lusitanus. As noted in an earlier section, Amatus spent 7 years in Antwerp before leaving for Italy in 1540 to become Professor of Medicine at Ferrara. Also Rodrigo de Castro, who was renowned for his text on diseases of women, came to Antwerp from Lisbon before going on to complete his illustrious career in Hamburg.

Luis Nunez, a colleague of Amatus left teaching posts at the Universities of Lisbon and Coimbra to established himself in Antwerp, where in 1545 he published a medical dictionary. Nunez also spent a period in Paris as physician to Catherine de Medici. Another of his famous patients was the Queen of England, whom he was called to treat in Brussels.

Another physician with the same name, Luiz Nunez II also was a noted scholar and author. He was the son of Alvaro Nunez, a physician who, in Peru, was burned at-the-stake in Lima in 1582.

Alvarez Nunez (Alvares Nouninus Hispanus) (d. 1603) had come to Antwerp as physician to Archduke Albert of Austria whom he accompanied from Lisbon. Remaining in Antwerp he gained a reputation for excellence as a physician, surgeon, and author.

Dionysis Rodrigues had been physician to the Queen of Portugal before first fleeing to London then settling in Antwerp in 1538. Two events were next in store for him—burning in effigy by the Inquisition in Lisbon and yet another move to Ferrara in Italy.

Hamburg

Hamburg's location at the western end of the Baltic-North Sea trade routes favored its development into a foremost port of the Hanseatic League of merchant cities. Its location was geographically intermediate between Scandinavia and the lands of the "New World". Additionally enhanced by protective fortifications, it assumed increasing importance as a trade center. Recognized as an imperial free city in 1510, Hamburg offered a freer atmosphere than did many contemporary European states.

When wealthy Spanish and Portuguese Marranos, who reached Hamburg in the late 1500's, were found to be observing Jewish customs, some of the citizenry sought their ouster. However, the City Council appreciated the economic benefits derived from the Jewish presence and negated moves for their expulsion. Marranos became increasingly involved in Hamburg's commercial activities as financiers, ship builders, skilled weavers, goldsmiths, and importers of sugar, tobacco, and coffee from the Spanish and Portuguese colonies. Moving into this favorable setting were physicians whose familiar family names identified their Spanish-Portuguese Jewish and Marrano heritages.

One of the best known and successful physicians was Rodrigo de Castro (1546-1627), whose noted medical treatises included a text on diseases of women. His vigorous work fighting an epidemic in Hamburg in 1596 resulted in a treatise on the nature and causes and methods of treatment and prevention of plague. First published in 1603, it was followed by several editions. Castro's son, Benedict (1597-1684), became physician to Queen Christina of Sweden.

Three physicians whose contributions were noted in the previous discussion of Holland also had Hamburg connections. Benjamin ben Immanuel Mussafia (Latin pen name of Dionysius) first entered practice in Hamburg and there in 1640, published his famous *Sacro-Medicae Sententiae ex Ribliis*. Jacob Hebraeus Rosales who had left Amsterdam for Hamburg, was made a Count Palatine in 1647 by Frederick III. Samuel de Silva, physician and literary antagonist of the philosopher da Costa, also spent some years of practice in Hamburg as well as in Holland.

England

At the time of the institution of the Spanish Inquisition and the expulsion of 1492, England's history of severe antiSemitism placed it outside the possibility of a refuge for fleeing Jews and Marranos. Series of hostile policies of the throne and acts of persecution and impoverishment culminated in Edward I's edict of banishment in 1290; all traces of an English Jewish populace were erased. During the reigns of Henry VIII (1509-1547) and Edward VI (1547-1553) the arrival of a small group of Marranos once again led to establishment of a settlement in London. However, this development did not last beyond the accession of Mary in 1553. The force of Catholic reaction during her reign led to another interruption of a Jewish presence. Then, with Elizabeth (1558-1603) on the throne, Jewish identity was resumed in London and Bristol, and in this development, physicians played major roles.

Of the Nunez family of physicians, Henrique Nunez spent 10 years in Bristol, where he also served as chief of its Jewish community before leaving for France in 1555. Hector Nunez, whose Spanish commercial connections were very useful to the English government, arrived in 1550 and 4 years later was elected a Fellow of both the Royal College of Physicians and the Royal College of Surgeons.

Roderigo Lopez, a physician and anatomist, was related through marriage to a noble who had connections with the English court. Thus, when Lopez fled from the Inquisition in 1559, appropriate introductions led to his becoming physician to Elizabeth I. However, 35 years later, he was charged with plotting against the Queen's life, sentenced, and executed in 1594.

Manuel Brudus was the son of Dionysus Brudus (1470–1540), a physician who had reached Antwerp and written important works on Galenic medicine and phlebotomy. Manuel, after practices in Venice and Flanders, ultimately came to England. His publications on diet in febrile diseases gained wide recognition.

By the early years of the 17th century, without a legal basis for existence, the Jewish presence in England faded. However, by mid years of the century, creation of more favorable conditions led to the re-emergence of a Marrano colony in London. With the ascendancy of Puritan doctrine and its respect for the Old Testament, Jews began to enjoy greater respect and tolerance. Additionally, the position of Oliver Cromwell became an important factor. Cromwell, aiming at increased commerce and economic advancement, sought to duplicate Holland and Turkey's model in which the roles of Marrano merchants and financiers were highly important in aiding their countries' progress.

In this new atmosphere conducive to Jewish resettlement, Ferdinand Mendez arrived in London in 1669 and 18 years later was admitted as a Fellow of the Royal College of Physicians. He became physician to Queen Catherine, attended King Charles II in his last illness, and introduced a new preparation into materia medica—Aqua de Ingleterra, (wine of quinine) derived from cinchona bark.

Isaac Abendana (1650–1710), was a descendent of Francisco Nunez Pereyra, who had changed his name to David Abendana after fleeing from Spain to Amsterdam. He studied medicine in Leyden and Cambridge and first became affiliated with academia in England in 1633 as librarian at Cambridge. He next taught at Trinity College and then in 1676 moved to Oxford as Reader in Hebrew Language and Literature.

Two prominent Marrano family names, Bueno and de Castro, again appear. Joseph Mendes Bueno served as a public physician in London during the second half of the 17th century and Jacob de Castro-Sacramento (1692–1762), after leaving Portugal, became a distinguished English physician and scientist.

The Colonies

The voyages of Christopher Columbus and Vasco da Gama offered new vistas to victims of the concurrent Inquisitions and expulsions in the very same countries represented by their exploring fleets. In emerging empires to the East and to the West, Marranos and exiled Jews seized the opportunity to explore possibilities for their shattered lives and livelihoods rebuilding.

Spanish America

Soon after Columbus' revelation of a "New World", it became apparent that the roots of man's inhumanity to man would and could be successfully transplanted to the newly encountered land. The concurrent events of 1492—Columbus' sighting of the Caribbean islands and the expulsion edict—were without meaning to the displaced because Spanish law prohibited professing Jews from living on any Spanish soil including its colonies. By decrees of the Spanish monarchs in 1501, prohibition of immigration to the Indies was added to the list of legal rights lost to any member of a family interrogated by the Inquisition. Within another 10 years, Queen Joan issued a decree in 1511 restricting all Marrano immigration to New Spain. Subsequently, Inquisitorial authority—given initially to friars and later to bishops—was extended to New Spain. The first Auto-da-Fé was held in Mexico City in 1528.

During the first half century of Spanish colonization relatively few cases of Judaizing were pursued and crypto-Jews actually practiced their faith little molested. However, local reaction to increasing immigration of Marranos triggered the establishment of an official Tribunal in 1572 (Fig. 8). With renewed activity of the Inquisition, even the conquistador Governor of Nuevo Leon, Luis de Carvajal, fell victim and in 1596 members of his crypto-Jewish family faced Autos-da-Fé and burning at-the-stake. Entering the 17th century, the Tribunal became more occupied with prosecuting a variety of heresy and morals offenders and as a result its attention was diverted from Judaizing activities. Then, in 1640, the situation again changed to the disadvantage of the crypto-Jews when the Duke of Braganca led Portugal's revolt against the rule of the King of Spain. Because the great majority of New Spain's crypto-Jews had Portuguese backgrounds or ancestry, they were affected by the backlash of this Iberian event and subjected to an escalation of persecution by the Inquisition.

Hordes' investigation (1980) of trial records of crypto-Jews in the Inquisition Section of the National Archives of Mexico uncovered the presence of practicing physicians in the Mexican crypto-Jewish community during the relatively tranquil interval period of the early to mid-17th century. Four were identified by name.

Pedro Tinoco planned to become a priest and studied grammar, rhetoric, and philosophy at the Universidad de Mexico, graduating in 1636. However, because of

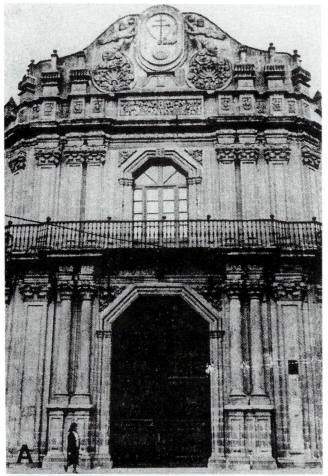

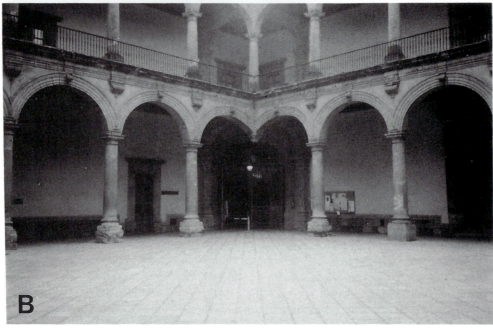

Figure 8. *Palacio de la Antigua Escuela de Medicina, Mexico City, Built in 1732–1737 to house the Mexican Tribunal of the Inquisition, showing the exterior front and the interior court where Inquisitorial trials were conducted (courtesy of Guy A. Settipane, M.D.).Before its construction, the Inquisition's activities were conducted in the convent of Santo Domingo and in neighboring houses. Following suspension of Inquisition in 1813, several sequential uses of the building included serving as the seat of the Marine and Army Tribunal and the government of the State of Mexico and housing of the first Lancasterian School of Mexico, the Councilar Seminary, and between 1854 and 1956 the Medical School of the National University of Mexico. Currently the restored building and its store of historic resources house the Museum of Medicine.*

the tenuous nature of a New Christian background, his maternal grandmother influenced him to study medicine instead. He was arrested by the Holy Office of the Inquisition in 1642, sentenced to exile at an Auto da Fé in 1649, and died the following year at age 29 en route to Veracruz.

Gaspar Nunez, a physician and surgeon of Mexico City, left for Cartagena in 1622 where he was known to practice in 1642.

Francisco Lopez Enriquez was a physician and surgeon for whom there were records of practice in Mexico City in 1622 and in Cartegena in 1642.

Rodrigo Fernandez Corres, born in Mexico City in 1623, was in the practice of medicine as of 1642, most likely in Veracruz.

In search of greater economic opportunities many of Mexico City's crypto-Jews left for other distant regions—e.g., the mining areas of Pachuca and the ports of Acapulco, Campeche, and Veracruz. Some went further, on to the Philippines.

In attempts to escape the Inquisition's renewed hunt for suspected secret Jews in the Spanish New World, many of Mexico's Marranos again went on the move and fled to land north of the Rio Grande. From records and artifacts, it may be assumed that current day New Mexico, rather than the East Coast British Colonies, was the first area in what now constitutes the continental United States to be entered by immigrants of Jewish descent. Within New Mexico's isolated mountain ranges, crypto-Jewish settlers apparently found protective refuge (Hordes). In addition to some traditional Jewish practices continued by overt Catholics, gravestones bearing both crosses and the six-point Star of David have been found in northern New Mexico cemeteries.

Although some immigration of crypto-Jews posing as Old Christians provided the nucleus of a slowly expanding Marrano population in Mexico, possibilities for their entries into the practice of medicine was closely monitored. Enforcement of a strict limpieza de sangra policy required proof of four ancestral generations of Catholic blood to qualify for a certificate of eligibility. Against this culturally restrictive and scientifically inhibiting background was the accomplishment of Ricardo Ossado, an Italian believed to be a Jew who escaped from Mexico. Ossado (c. 1647) published *El Libro del Judio*, a compendium of Maya herbs, medicines, and diseases; it became a reference text which found continued use for almost 300 years.

In 1570 the Inquisition was established in Peru and its first Auto-da-Fé was held in Lima 3 years later. Among those burned at-the-stake were the physicians Juan Alvarez in 1580 and Alvaro Nunez of La Plata, Argentina, in 1582. In 1610 New Granada later known as Colombia, initiated the Inquisition; the conduct of a

tribunal in Cartegena and a series of Autos-da-Fés soon followed.

In Chile, a highly distinguished New World physician fell victim to the Inquisition. Francisco Maldonado de Silva (1592–1639), also a poet and philosopher of "New Christian" parentage, was convicted of Judaizing and was held in a dungeon. Keeping faithful to his beliefs, during imprisonment he even converted two Catholics to Judaism. After 12 years de Silva was taken to Peru for further punishment and burned at-the-stake at an Auto-da-Fé in Lima.

Ultimately, the Peace of Westphalia in 1648, which ended Europe's 30 Years' War, forced Spain to concede to Holland, England, and France freedom of the seas and temporary rights of settlement in the West Indies. Accordingly, the door to immigration to the New World then opened for Jews of Spanish-Portuguese origin who earlier had found refuge in those three countries.

Portuguese America/Brazil

In 1502, 2 years after Portugal's Admiral Pedro Alvares Cabral landed on the coast of what is now Brazil, a consortium of New Christians received a franchise from King Manoel to colonize and exploit the newly founded possession. They soon became engaged in the business of exporting brazilwood as the source of textile dye. That fleeing Jews also might find refuge in Brazil, however, was ruled out as a possibility as early as 1508. Coincident with the decree of expulsion, Portugal followed the lead of Spanish law and also took steps to enforce the exclusion of professing Jews from its New World colony.

By 1548 immigrating Marranos were responsible for the beginning of a sugar industry; they had brought cane from Madeira and after its successful transplantation, developed sugar plantations and mills. As Marranos became prominent and prospered, the force of the Church once again was used against them by envious and zealous fellow settlers. In 1567 the Portuguese Regent issued an edict forbidding further Marrano settlement in Brazil. However, 10 years later, on payment of a large sum by Marranos of Lisbon and Brazil, a repealing edict was issued and privileges of residence and commerce were granted.

Although a formal structure for the Inquisition was never set up in Brazil, one aspect of the practice did impact on the role of Jews in the country's development. New Christians, who were reported by spies and denounced or even suspected of being secret Jews, were seized and sent to Lisbon to stand trial. After Spain, under Philip II, seized Portugal in 1580 this practice was strengthened by periodic official Church Inquisitorial commissions. At the same time, by a curious scheme of interchanging two-way traffic, one form of punishment for relapsed Marranos convicted of Judaizing was banishment to Portugal. Additionally diverting, Spain's rather tenuous hold on its new Portuguese colony prevented rigid enforcement of Spanish law in Brazil.

By the end of the first decade of the 17th century, Jewish physicians were in practice in the capital city of Bahia. They were also among those who were victims of the policy of persecution which had been extended to Brazil. Father and son physicians, Abraham and David Raphael de Mercado, were forced to leave the country in 1655, and Manoel Mendes Monforte in 1723, was brought back to Lisbon for punishment by the Inquisition.

On the brighter side of Brazil's story was the role of The Netherlands' involvement in colonizing. From the time Holland made its first attempts at the conquest of Brazil in the second decade of the 17th century, the Jews were friendly and helpful to Holland's ambitions. In 1621 the Jews of Amsterdam contributed to the establishment of the Dutch West Indies Company and some were members of the company's directorate.

Unfortunately plans for promoting Dutch interests in Bahia after its capture in 1624 came to a halt the next year when the Portuguese retook the city. Seven years later, the Dutch in 1631 captured Recife (Pernambuco) and Bahia's Jews moved into the city with them. However, once again freedom, prosperity and the opportunity for pursuit of professions came to an end in 1654; Portugal was finally victorious in the guerilla war in which the Jews fought alongside their Dutch benefactors. Capitulation to the Portuguese brought another edict of expulsion for the Jews along with their fellow Dutch. Many of the captured were sent to Lisbon for trial as Marrano Judaizers; others with Jews, who were not hanged as traitors, returned to Holland. Still others would be welcomed into new opportunities in Holland's Caribbean colonies—Caracas, Cayenne, St. Thomas, and New Amsterdam (later renamed New York).

East India

The establishment of Goa as the seat of Portugal's Viceroy of India in 1510 offered opportunities for fleeing Spanish and Portuguese Jews, Marranos, and other New Christians who might wish to turn to Judaizing. Pioneering work in the Portuguese East Indies gained fame for two Marrano physicians, Garcia de Orta and Crustoval d'Acosta.

Orta left a professorship of logic at Lisbon, and in 1534 sailed to India where he traveled and studied the country and its flora. He became a pioneer in the study of tropical diseases and in the founding of botanical science. His collection and study of Oriental medicinal plants published in 1563 as *Colloquies dos Simplex Drogas e Cosao Medicines de India* was the first and most important contribution on the subject introduced to European medicine. It was translated into five languages and appeared in several editions during the next 4 centuries. Orta was referred to as the most illustrious representative of the natural sciences.

The large influx of successful Jewish and Marrano immigrants to Goa again brought forth the Church's expression of hate. In mid-16th century ecclesiastic authorities sought to bring the Inquisition to Goa and ultimately established it in 1560 (Fig. 9). Not even Orta's death in 1568 could escape the Inquisition's effects. Twelve years later in a posthumous trial, Orta was convicted as a suspected Jew and his body was exhumed and burned.

Orta's studies were extended by Acosta, a Marrano born in Mozambique to where his parents had fled from Spain. As a physician and botanist, he did research on the native medicinal plants and drugs. Acosta lived and traveled in India and the Middle East and in 1578 he published *Tractado de las Drogas*, an enlargement of Orta's work.

While the promising Jewish settlement in Portuguese Goa ultimately suffered and disappeared, by contrast the Jews in Dutch India fared remarkably well. On the

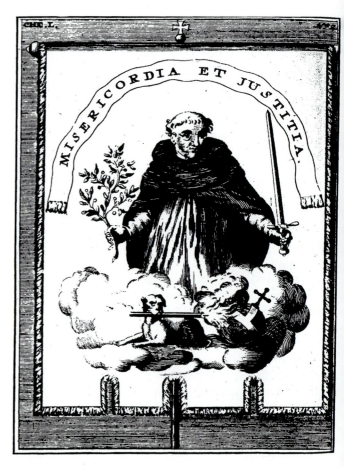

Figure 9. *Banner of the Inquisition of Goa (Osterreichische National Bibliothek, Picture Archives, Vienna).*

Malabar coast, they were protected and granted freedom of worship and cultural autonomy by native rejas. Between 1663 and 1795, under Dutch rule and in close bond with the Amsterdam community, many Jewish immigrants came from Spain, Portugal, North Africa, Germany, Persia, Palestine, Syria, Iraq, and provinces of the Ottoman Empire. In Cochin they prospered as merchants and agents and in careers as diplomats and physicians.

British Colonies

In addition to providing a new country of cultural and economic opportunities, England offered access to involvements and developments taking shape in its emerging colonial empire. In contrast to policies in Spanish and Portuguese America where Jews were ruled undesirable, they were welcomed to British Jamaica and Barbados. There they helped to create the sugar industry as they had done for Brazil. When forced to leave Portuguese Brazil with the expulsion, the physicians Abraham de Mercado and his son David Raphael Mercado were among the first authorized by Oliver Cromwell to settle in Barbados in 1655.

The first Jewish physician to reach the North American colonies was Jacob Lumbrozo, a native of Lisbon, who arrived in 1656. One of the earliest practitioners in Maryland, he developed a successful practice in Charles County where he was known as the "Jew Doctor". Until his death in 1666 Lumbrozo played an important role in the county's economic activities.

Sixty-seven years after Lumbrozo's arrival, a second Jewish physician immigrated to colonial America from Lisbon. In 1733, 1 year after the founding of Georgia, Samuel Nunez Ribiero reached Savannah. Governor James Oglethorpe praised Ribiero's care of the sick, commended him to the trustees of the Colony, and gave him a land grant in gratitude for the dedicated services he rendered during a raging epidemic.

At about the same time another Portuguese physician named Siccari entered practice in Virginia. Thomas Jefferson, in speaking of Siccari, credited him with introducing tomatoes into America and with advocating the health benefits to be derived from the tomato as a dietary item. It was important in this regard for misconceptions to be overcome; for many years the tomato had been considered poisonous and of use only as a garden ornament.

In 1744 Isaac Cohen arrived in Lancaster, Pennsylvania, from Hamburg. On entering practice he announced his intent to cure gratis any poor person who presented a certificate from a clergyman.

Early records of New York reveal physician members of the first Spanish—Portuguese Jewish congregation. In 1742 there was one physician with the Sephardic name of Nunez and another Elias Woolin, a native of Bohemia. Physician Jacob Levy arrived from Germany in 1750, and in 1761 Andrew Judah came from Holland and subsequently moved to South Carolina.

With the Declaration of Independence in 1776 and the surrender of the British army in 1783, emergence of the United States of America from the English Colonies initiated even greater opportunities to seek new lives supported by beliefs in the human values of freedom and safety. During the next century, a steady stream of immigrants crossed the Atlantic. Among these, an ever increasing number of Jewish physicians were added to the roles of contributors to clinical care and the advancement of medical teaching and research in America. How appropriate that those fleeing from oppression and persecution, so typified by the horrors and tragedies of the era of Spanish—Portuguese victimization, would one day be welcomed to the harbor of New York with the words of an American of Sephardic Jewish heritage.

Give me your tired, your poor,
Your huddled masses yearning to breathe free,
The wretched refuse of your teeming shore,
Send these, the homeless, tempest-tossed, to me;
I lift my lamp beside the golden door.
Emma Lazarus (1849–1887); from the *New Colossus* (1883); inscribed in 1886 on a bronze plaque, placed inside the base of the Statue of Liberty.

COMMENTARY

"What excellent fools Religion makes of men!
"Ben Jonson, *Seganus*, Act 1 (1603)

Skills, talents, and knowledge which owed their origins to Iberia's Golden Age thus were seeded to other lands and cultures. The sources of these transplanted activities and contributions, if retained and nurtured, might have prevented Spain and Portugal's precipitous decline from the social and professional forefront of medicine and scholarly pursuits. Especially pertinent to these examples was the observation of the Turkish Sultan Bajazet. How could Ferdinand be considered a wise king, Bajazet noted, when he impoverished Spain and enriched Turkey.

Spanish royalty had only to look within the confines of its own court to perceive what the country's future in medicine might have been. At the height of the Inquisition's frenzy, a Castilian Marrano physician rose to the pinnacle of fame. Ludovicus Mercatus/Luiz Mercado (1513–1600) (Fig. 10), who held the rank of First Professor of Medicine at the University of Valladolid, was celebrated as the most brilliant physician of his period; he was chosen to be physician-in-chief to Philip II, King of Spain, Portugal, Naples, and Sicily (1590–1598), and to Philip II's successor Philip III (1598–1621). Renown as a clinician and prolific author, he

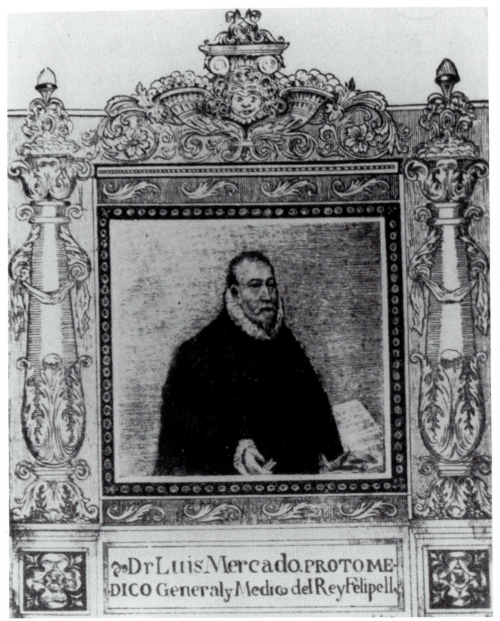

Figure 10. *Ludovicus Mercatus/Luiz Mercado (circa 1513–1600); from the Frontispiece of his* El Libro de la Peste *(courtesy of National Library of Medicine).*

wrote on fevers, infectious maladies, plaque, diseases of women and children, and heredity. His portrait by El Greco was placed in the Prado in Madrid. After Luiz, the family name of Mercado in scattered fashion appeared in Hamburg, Amsterdam, and Brazil.

Through self-inflicted loss, the monarchs of Spain and Portugal had contributed to advances in distant countries and continents. How tragic was the cost for the innocent subjects of Spanish-Portuguese orchestration. (To be concluded)

BIBLIOGRAPHY

Dale PM. Christopher Columbus. In Medical Biographies, The Ailments of Thirty-three Famous Persons. Norman, University of Oklahoma Press, 1952, pp. 16–19.

Encyclopaedia Judaica. Vol II, Medicine. Jerusalem, Keter Publishing House, 1971, pp. 1178–1196.

Friedenwald H. The Jews and Medicine, Essays. Baltimore: Johns Hopkins Press, 1944.

Fuson RH. The Log of Christopher Columbus (transl). Camden, ME: International Marine Publishing Co, 1987.

Grangel LS, Palermo JR. Medicina y sociedad en la espana renacentista. In: Historia Universal de la Medicina. Entralgo PL, ed. Barcelona: Salvat Editores, 1973, pp. 181–189.

Chapter 16

Portugal's Contribution to Navigation and Discovery of the New World

Manuel Luciano da Silva, M.D.

ABSTRACT

Even before the birth of Prince Henry the Navigator (1394) Portugal had displayed a maritime calling due to its 500-mile shore line and numerous natural bays. Inspired by the riches of India he saw during the Portuguese exploration along the coast of West Africa, Prince Henry set out methodically to collect information by bringing together Jews and Moors with geographical knowledge to found his School of Navigation. From 1415 until his death in 1460 he attracted to his school the foremost contemporary scholars in mathematics, astronomy, and cartography along with experts in knowledge of the compass, astrolabe, water currents, and the winds. This concentration of talent yielded the invention of the caravel, the most important navigational advancement of the time, crucial for long voyages across the high seas. Although the rest of Europe busied itself in political and religious wars, for 70 years (1415–1492) Portugal alone pursued the discovery of the Atlantic. "No nation in the 15th century exhibited so great a spirit of maritime enterprise as the Portuguese."[1]

About 2,389 years ago in Athens, Plato, the great Greek philosopher, founded his School of Philosophy called "Academia" because he held his classes in a garden named "Academus." His pupils were called peripatetic because they walked around the garden.

Manuel Luciano da Silva investigates the history of discoveries and is president of the Bristol County Medical Center, Bristol, R.I.

Today, we do not find any vestiges of Plato's School but nobody doubts its existence.

Aristotle, Plato's most famous student, began his School of Philosophy 2,339 years ago, also in Athens, in a garden called "Lyceum," a name used even today to designate high schools in many countries. There are no vestiges of Aristotle's "Lyceum" but nobody doubts its existence.

In 1418, 574 years ago, Prince Henry of Portugal founded his School of Navigation, at the Promontory of Sagres (Sacred Rock), the most southwestern point of Portugal. Today, we still see the buildings of the School of Navigation and the giant Rose Compass on its campus confirming that indeed his Nautical School existed!

Even before Prince Henry was born, (1394) Portugal had already shown a maritime vocation due to its long shore (500 miles) and natural bays. King Dinis had founded the Portuguese Navy in 1317. The same Monarch ordered the large Leiria pine forest to be sown so that the kingdom could be supplied with enough wood for naval construction. He also founded Coimbra University in 1290 and nationalized the Order of Templars converting them into the Portuguese Order of Christ. These developments created the setting that led Portugal to conduct her sea explorations.

The greatest desire of all the noble Princes of Portugal, as in the rest of Europe, was to receive the rites of knighthood on the battlefield. King John I once planned a tournament with pennants and fanfare to be held in Lisbon (c. 1412). Here, his three sons, Dom Duarte (later King), Dom Pedro (the Traveler) and Dom Henrique (the Navigator), were to be knighted after participating in mock warfare begun at the end of

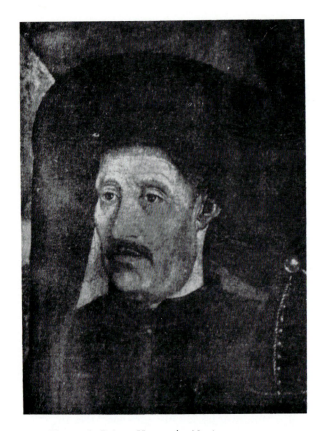

Figure 1. Prince Henry the Navigator.

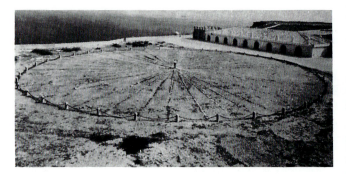

Figure 3. Rose Compass on the grounds of the School of Navigation.

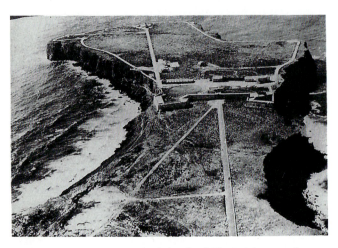

Figure 2. Prince Henry's School of Navigation at Sagres, Portugal.

a pompous ceremony. But, the young Princes preferred to fight in real combat rather than take part in "festas" or accept invitations to socialize. To satisfy the wishes of his sons, who insisted on proving themselves in battle, King John I proposed an alternative. He suggested the idea of a strong attack on Granada, the Moorish Kingdom bordering Algarve, which was a perpetual affront to the Christians. The King's advisors, and his young and restless sons finally persuaded him to conquer instead, the Moorish City of Ceuta near Gibraltar, which was the principal haunt of pirates and a constant hindrance to commerce between the Mediterranean and the Atlantic.

CEUTA

The preparations for the armada to Ceuta took 3 years to complete (1412–1415). There was a general mobilization. Despite all the ongoing naval construction and military preparations the destination of the armada was kept a secret. On August 21, 1415, with a fleet of 200 vessels and 20,000 men, the Portuguese captured Ceuta, a City "rich and opulent, full of every luxury in precious markets." (2)

Thus, the young Princes became Knights in Africa. The news of the capture of Ceuta caused a tremendous sensation throughout the Christian world. But more important, it gave Prince Henry the inspiration to create a school of navigation aimed at obtaining directly from India, the ivory, spices, and riches he had seen in Ceuta. Upon returning from Ceuta, Prince Henry decided to collect methodically, all the valuable information concerning the mysteries of the Moslem World. For this, he "brought to Lisbon many Jews and Moors with the knowledge of the remote provinces, and the coasts and seas contiguous to them." (2) In the meantime, Infante Dom Pedro had traveled throughout Europe collecting nautical information and establishing diplomatic contacts that proved to be quite beneficial to the discoveries.

From 1415 until his death in 1460—married to the idea of sea exploration—Prince Henry invited and attracted to his School of Navigation, situated first in Lisbon, and later in Sagres, the foremost scholars in mathematics, astronomy, cartography, and those that were experts regarding the encompass, the astrolabe, water currents, and the winds. Pooling together and applying all this theoretical knowledge, the most important practical accomplishment of Prince Henry's School of Navigation was the invention of the caravel.

The acquisition of the caravel eliminated the problem of feeding the large crew in the galley-type ships and allowed navigators to make long voyages across the high seas. By reducing the size of the crew considerably, more food could be stored and longer voyages made possible. The caravel was the first ship used by man that could tack against the wind.

Prince Henry spent his entire fortune to maintain his school. He exhausted the coffers of the rich Order of Christ, but never diminished in his perseverance while urging his captains to explore further into the unknown seas. The Villa do Infante (Prince Henry's Town) was specially built as the campus of the School of Navigation. The style of campus buildings is characteristic of Northern Portugal where Prince Henry was born and does not follow the Algarve architecture.

THE FEARSOME CAPE

With the return of Gil Eanes in 1434, after having passed the Cape of Bojador, or Fearsome Cape, the cold reasoning and scientific knowledge of Prince Henry had finally triumphed. Gone were the superstitions and legends of boiling oceans and dark sinister seas with monsters that haunted humanity for centuries. When Prince Henry died, his sailors had already reached the Gulf of Guinea near the Equator. By this time they had sailed beyond the site of the North Star, which had guided their ships in the North Atlantic, but they encountered the constellation of the Southern Cross where the South Star served to orient their course through the South Atlantic, around the Cape of Good Hope.

Never before in the history of mankind had a civilization gone through so many large scale changes as during the period of the discoveries. Europe was brought into contact, for the first time, with strange civilizations, new races, and unknown islands. Huge Continents, vast oceans, and even constellations never seen before by the Europeans were discovered.

Very few men had such an impact on the history of the world as Prince Henry. He had the foresight to form his Nautical School at Sagres and make it the scientific center of the world, thereby launching: "Humanity's first systematic work in the scientific of exploration." (3)

THE MEANING OF DISCOVERY

Many historians have continually misused the verb "to discover." They imply that discovery is a one-way street. It is not. Discovery involves a two-way traffic. (2)

If a ship set sail from Europe for the precise purpose of discovering unknown land and never returns, nothing would be discovered. Even if it arrives at new lands and the crew lives happily ever after but were unable

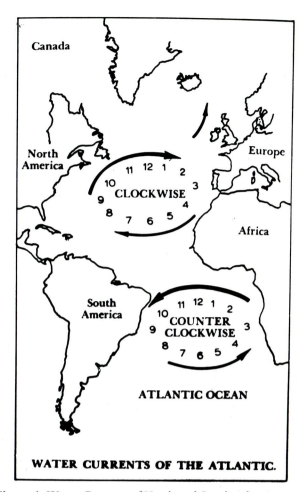

Figure 4. *Water Currents of North and South Atlantic.*

to return to Europe to actually tell of their findings, no discovery would have been accomplished. We have always been able to observe the moon and other planets. Yet until recently, we were not able to discover them because we did not have the means to send an astronaut to explore them and report back to earth. To discover, i.e., setting out and reporting back, represents a stage of civilization that was first initiated in a scientific manner by Prince Henry's School of Navigation. No one should dare to speak about maritime discoveries without first studying thoroughly the water currents and the winds of the Atlantic.

WATER CURRENTS AND THE WINDS

The Canary Current originates at the Promontory of Sagres where Prince Henry situated his school, and runs parallel to the African coast. It continues north of the Cape Verde Islands, and becomes the North Equatorial Current, or Trade Winds, crossing the Atlantic parallel to the equator and emptying into the Caribbean Sea. Then, the Gulf Stream, like a huge river, flows toward Europe and at the Azores branches out into the North Atlantic Current and the Canary Current. This

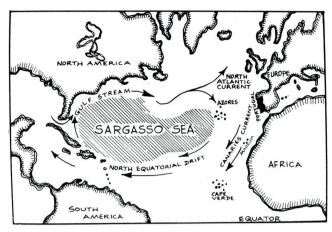

Figure 5. Sargasso Sea, the Heart of the Atlantic.

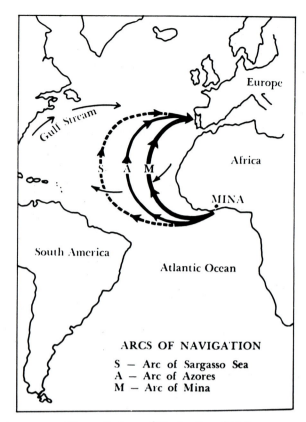

ARCS OF NAVIGATION
S — Arc of Sargasso Sea
A — Arc of Azores
M — Arc of Mina

Figure 6. Arcs of Navigation, SAM.

dance of the Atlantic has not changed for thousands of years. All these currents create boundaries around the vast sea of seaweed, a sea without shores, forming the heart of the Atlantic. The Portuguese call it Sargasso Sea, a maritime name that is internationally known.

Benjamin Franklin was the first since the Portuguese navigators to recognize the navigational importance of the Atlantic Currents. As a Deputy Postmaster of the colonies, Franklin took an interest in the currents that cold increase the sailing speed of the mail ship to Europe. For this purpose, Franklin had the first chart of the Gulf Stream made. (1769)

However, the first modern oceanographic studies of the currents and winds in the Atlantic were carried out by Prince Albert of Monaco (1885–1887). By throwing different sized bottles and barrels into various points in the North Atlantic, he proved that all these buoys made a circle surrounding the Sargasso Sea and that all of them were carried toward the American Continent by the Trade Winds or North Equatorial drift. He also proved that none of the objects crossed the Equator into the South Atlantic. The findings of Prince Albert have been confirmed by the Woods Hole Oceanographic Institute of Massachusetts.

The Gulf Stream has always brought strange objects to shores of the Azores and Portugal from the New World. Vegetable matter, pine trunks, (Azores had no pine trees) and canoes served as evidence to the navigators that unknown lands lay further west.

NAVIGATIONAL ARCS

One fundamental method of navigating under sail is to travel in an arc, or great circle. During the first period (1416–1434) of the discoveries, the navigators were reluctant to venture too far into the open seas, until in 1434, they passed the Cape of Bojador in Africa. Sailing out from Lisbon toward the African coast was fairly easy because they followed the Canary current

and winds. Returning to Portugal, they were forced to make a broad swing at considerable distance away from the coast. On each voyage they sailed in ever-widening arms westward into the open Atlantic taking advantage of the Canary winds, now at their right (first part of the navigational arc) and then joined the Gulf Stream to Continental Portugal (second half of the navigational arc). With this technique, the navigators continued to make a series of wider navigational arcs, establishing the now conventional sailing routes: (1) Arc of Mina (present day Ghana), (2) Arc of Azores, and (3) Arc of Sargasso Sea.

In 1537, Pedro Nunes, a Portuguese navigator and mathematician, printed the first details of navigational arcs, or great-circle routes. The discovery of the Sargasso Sea and the western-most islands of the Azores was made on return voyages from Africa. Soon the Portuguese pilots learned that navigating the high seas was much easier than sailing along the coast where the water currents and the winds did not follow a fixed pattern. The North Atlantic became their University of Navigation. The Madeira, Azorean, Canary, and Cape Verde Islands became the "interplanetary stations," the stepping stones in the discovery of the unknown continents.

The knowledge acquired by the Portuguese during the first open-sea voyages in the North Atlantic gave

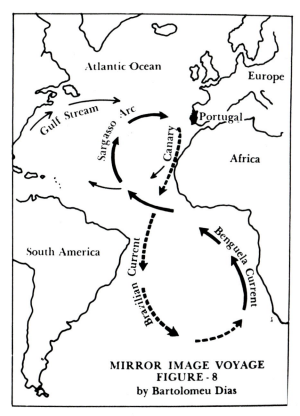

Figure 7. Mirror Image Voyage, Figure 8.

them the key with which, from discovery to discovery, with method and perseverance, they could also open the doors of the South Atlantic Ocean. It was Bartolomeu Dias, the master of the caravel, who passed the Cape of Good Hope in 1487 because he realized that he could not navigate against the Guinea current. Instead he decided to take a southwesterly course (Brazilian Current), out into the open sea, in search of a more favorable wind. His voyage was a mirror image in the South Atlantic of the Sargasso Navigational Route in the North Atlantic.

Sailing in an arc had already solved many problems in the North Atlantic during Prince Henry's lifetime. On his return, Bartolomeu Dias followed the Benguela Current, parallel to the African Coast, and sailed toward the equator, continuing along the conventional Sargasso-Azores Route to Lisbon. His great achievement was first in being able to complete the gigantic figure-8 water route embracing both Atlantics.

Even today, many scholars who know nothing about nautical science are amazed to learn that Vasco da Gama in his first voyage to India followed the Brazilian Current. This current, which comprised the southwest arc of the figure-8 water route, led him to the Indian Ocean. The Corte Real family of navigators were familiar with the technique of sailing in an arc long before Bartolomeu Dias or Vasco da Gama. Since 1472, when John Vaz Corte Real returned from discovering New-

foundland, for which he was rewarded with the governorship of half the Island of Terceira, the Corte Real family spent all its energies pursuing the Northwest passage to India. Thus, from the Island of Terceira, the Portuguese navigators reached North America by sailing in a Northwest arc which cut across the Gulf Stream. They made their return voyage by joining the main current of the Gulf Stream leading them directly to the Azores.

The more knowledge we have of the oceanic forces—water currents and winds—that once moved the caravels across the Atlantic the more convinced we become that the discovery of the water route to America—North and South—was, indeed, forced upon the Portuguese navigators and therefore the easiest of all the discoveries.

It is noteworthy that although Europe was involved in political and religious wars, Portugal for more than 70 years (1415—1492) was pursuing the discovery of the Atlantic alone. When the other nations in Europe became aware of the importance of the Portuguese achievements, they attempted to compete in the race for discoveries but were never able to surpass the experience nor offset the advantage that the Portuguese sailors had acquired during their many years of maritime exploration. By the time the Portuguese passed the Cape of Good Hope in 1487, they had already gained such a momentum of knowledge of navigating the high seas, that no other nation was able to reach their level of scientific navigation.

Portugal had pilots not only for her own needs, but enough to give away. In order to carry out their maritime enterprises, other nations were forced to recruit among the experienced Portuguese masters (e.g., Estevão Gomes, Fernão de Magalhães (Magellan) and João

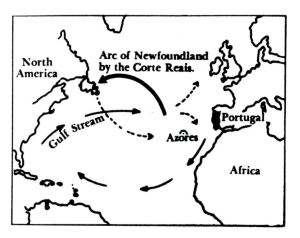

Figure 8. Arch of Newfoundland by Corte Reais.

Cabrilho). Suffice to say that all five Spanish ships in Magellan's fleet were piloted by Portuguese navigators.

There is a striking similarity between the Portuguese discoverers of the Prince Henry School of Navigation at Sagres and the American astronauts of the Outer Space Explorations at Cape Kennedy. The American astronauts picked up where the Portuguese navigators left off on humanity's constant exploration of our Universe.

REFERENCES

1. Harrisse, Henry. *The Discovery of North America*. In: A Critical, Documentary and Historical Investigation. Amsterdam North Israel: 1969, First Published London-Paris: 1892, p. 51
2. Da Silva, Manuel Luciano. *Portuguese Pilgrims and Dighton Rock*. Nelson D. Martins, Ed. Bristol, R. I. May 1971, Chapters 3 & 4.
3. Larsen, Sofus. *The Discovery of North American Twenty Years Before Columbus*. Cophenhagen: Levin & Munksgaard Publishers, 1925, p. 5.   □

Index

(Page numbers followed by "t" inicates material from a table)